MECHANISMS OF LYMPHOCYTE ACTIVATION AND IMMUNE REGULATION II

ADVANCES IN EXPERIMENTAL MEDICINE AND BIOLOGY

Recent Volumes in this Series

Volume 249
MINERAL ABSORPTION IN THE MONOGASTRIC GI TRACT:
Chemical, Nutritional, and Physiological Aspects
Edited by Frederick R. Dintzis and Joseph A. Laszlo

Volume 250
PROGRESS IN POLYAMINE RESEARCH:
Novel Biochemical, Pharmacological, and Clinical Aspects
Edited by Vincenzo Zappia and Anthony E. Pegg

Volume 251
IMMUNOBIOLOGY OF PROTEINS AND PEPTIDES V: Vaccines—Mechanism, Design, and Applications
Edited by M. Zouhair Atassi

Volume 252
DRUGS, SYSTEMIC DISEASES, AND THE KIDNEY
Edited by Alberto Amerio, Pasquale Coratelli, Vito M. Campese, and Shaul G. Massry

Volume 253A
PURINE AND PYRIMIDINE METABOLISM IN MAN VI, Part A:
Clinical and Molecular Biology
Edited by Kiyonobu Mikanagi, Kusuki Nishioka, and William N. Kelley

Volume 253B
PURINE AND PYRIMIDINE METABOLISM IN MAN VI, Part B:
Basic Research and Experimental Biology
Edited by Kiyonobu Mikanagi, Kusuki Nishioka, and William N. Kelley

Volume 254
MECHANISMS OF LYMPHOCYTE ACTIVATION AND IMMUNE REGULATION II
Edited by Sudhir Gupta and William E. Paul

Volume 255
CALCIUM PROTEIN SIGNALING
Edited by H. Hidaka

Volume 256
ENDOTOXIN
Edited by Herman Friedman, T. W. Klein, Masayasu Nakano, and Alois Nowotny

---

A Continuation Order Plan is available for this series. A continuation order will bring delivery of each new volume immediately upon publication. Volumes are billed only upon actual shipment. For further information please contact the publisher.

MECHANISMS OF LYMPHOCYTE ACTIVATION AND IMMUNE REGULATION II

Edited by

Sudhir Gupta

University of California, Irvine
Irvine, California

and

William E. Paul

National Institute of Allergy and Infectious Diseases
National Institutes of Health
Bethesda, Maryland

SPRINGER SCIENCE+BUSINESS MEDIA, LLC

Library of Congress Cataloging in Publication Data

International Conference on Lymphocyte Activation and Immune Regulation (2nd: 1988: Newport Beach, Calif.)
Mechanisms of lymphocyte activation and immune regulation II / edited by Sudhir Gupta and William E. Paul.
p. cm. – (Advances in experimental medicine and biology; v. 254)
"Proceedings of the Second International Conference on Lymphocyte Activation and Immune Regulation, held February 18–20, 1988, in Newport Beach, California" – T.p. verso.
Includes bibliographies and index.
ISBN 978-1-4757-5805-4 ISBN 978-1-4757-5803-0 (eBook)
DOI 10.1007/978-1-4757-5803-0
1. Lymphocyte transformation – Congresses. 2. Immune response – Regulation – Congresses. I. Gupta, Sudhir. II. Paul, William E. III. Title. IV. Title: Mechanisms of lymphocyte activation and immune regulation 2. V. Series.
[DNLM: 1. Lymphocyte Transformation – congresses. 2. Lymphocytes – immunology – congresses. 3. Lymphocytes – physiology – congresses. WH 200 I572m 1988]
QR185.8.L9I553 1988
616.07′9 – dc20
DNLM/DLC 89-16125
for Library of Congress CIP

Proceedings of the Second International Conference on Lymphocyte Activation and Immune Regulation held February 18–20, 1988, in Newport Beach, California

Originally published by Plenum Press, New York in 1989
Softcover reprint of the hardcover 1st edition 1989

CONTRIBUTORS

PAMELA J. BJORKMAN--Department of Medical Microbiology, Stanford University School of Medicine, Stanford, California 94305

MICHAEL B. BRENNER--Laboratory of Immunochemistry, Dana Farber Cancer Institute, Boston, Massachusetts 02115

MICHAEL D. CAHALAN--Department of Physiology and Biophysics, University of California, Irvine, California 92717

KATHRYN CALAME--Department of Microbiology, Columbia University College of Physicians and Surgeons, New York, New York 1003

MARK M. DAVIS--Department of Medical Microbiology, Stanford University School of Medicine, Stanford, California 94305

ANTHONY DeFRANCO--Departments of Microbiology and Immunology and Biochemistry and Biophysics, University of California, San Francisco, California 94143

CHARLES A. DINARELLO--Department of Medicine, Tufts University School of Medicine and New England Medical Center Hospital, Boston, Massachusetts 02111

WARNER C. GREENE--Howard Hughes Medical Institute, Duke University Medical Center, Durham, North Carolina 27710

SUDHIR GUPTA--Division of Basic and Clinical Immunology, University of California, Irvine, California 92717

JOHN H. KEHRL--Laboratory of Immunoregulation, National Institutes of Allergy and Infectious Diseases, National Institutes of Health, Bethesda, Maryland 20892

PAUL W. KINCADE--Oklahoma Medical Research Foundation, Oklahoma City, Oklahoma 73104

TADAMITSU KISHIMOTO--Institute for Molecular and Cellular Biology, Osaka University, Osaka 565, Japan

GERRY G.B. KLAUS--National Institute for Medical Research, London, United Kingdom

RICHARD KLAUSNER--National Institute of Child Health and Human Development, National Institutes of Health, Bethesda, Maryland 20892

FRITZ MELCHERS--Basel Institute for Immunology, Basel, Switzerland

RICHARD J. ROBB--Medical Products Department, E.I. du Pont de Nemours & Co., Glenolden, Pennsylvania 19036

EVA SEVERINSON--Department of Immunology, Stockholm University, Stockholm, Sweden

ARTHUR WEISS--Departments of Medicine and of Microbiology and Immunology, Howard Hughes Medical Institute, University of California, San Francisco, California 94143

PREFACE

The activation of lymphocytes by physiologic ligands has become a central area of study for immunologists. Furthermore, lymphocytes offer many advantages for the study of general aspects of receptor-mediated cellular activation. For these reasons, research on the cellular and molecular aspects of the activation of lymphocytes by antigens, antigen analogues, lymphokines and other growth factors has expanded enormously in the last several years. A series of conferences, "The International Conferences on Lymphocyte Activation", has been initiated to meet the growing need for a forum for the discussion of the topics that are included within the area of lymphocyte activation.

This volume represents the proceedings of the Second International Conference on Lymphocyte Activation and Immune Regulation, held on February 18-20, 1988 at Newport Beach, California. The proceedings comprise four major sections. The first deals with the T cell receptors and T cell activation. It includes a model for the T cell receptor interaction with a complex of MHC plus antigen, structure of $\gamma\delta$ T cell receptor and their distinct isotypic forms, the role of zeta chain in the expression and structure of T cell receptors and its role in transmembrane signalling. The use of somatic cell mutants in the study of signal transduction function of the T cell antigen receptors and the early and late steps of signal transduction via α/β T cell antigen receptors are discussed. The second section presents the structures and functions of interleukin 1 and interleukin 2 and their receptors. The third section includes B cell development and B cell activation. The cellular and molecular requirements for B cell lymphopoiesis and the factors that bind to functionally important regions of IgH chain promotor and enhancer are presented. The pool of precursor B lymphocytes using monoclonal antibodies and precursor B cell specific genes has been identified. A role of G protein and membrane ion channels in signal transduction of human and murine B cells is discussed in detail. The fourth section includes the role of interleukins 4, 5, 6 in the B cell activation, proliferation and differentiation. A role of interleukin 6 in the immunopathogenesis of autoimmune disorders is discussed. Data are presented for various effects of transforming growth factor on B cell proliferation and differentiation, including interactions with other cytokines. This book should be of interest to researchers in basic immunology and molecular biology.

Sudhir Gupta
William E. Paul

CONTENTS

T CELL RECEPTORS AND T CELL ACTIVATION

INTERLEUKIN 1 AND INTERLEUKIN 2 RECEPTORS

B LYMPHOCYTE DEVELOPMENT AND B CELL ACTIVATION

INTERLEUKINS AND B LYMPHOCYTE ACTIVATION

T CELL RECEPTORS AND T CELL ACTIVATION

A MODEL FOR T CELL RECEPTOR AND MHC/PEPTIDE INTERACTION

Mark M. Davis[*#] and Pamela J. Bjorkman[#]

The Howard Hughes Medical Institute[*] and
Department of Medical Microbiology[#]
Stanford University School of Medicine
Stanford, CA

INTRODUCTION

For some time it has been known that T cell recognition of antigen occurs in an MHC restricted fashion (1-3). Much recent evidence suggests that the antigens 'seen' by T cell receptors (TcR) are fragments (presumably derived by intracellular processing) bound to MHC molecules at a single site (4-10) By contrast, the immunoglobulin (Ig) B cell receptor can bind to native antigen alone. Structurally and genetically however, both immunoglobulins and T cell receptors seem very similar. Both are derived from the relatively random juxtaposition of different coding segments (V, D and J) of DNA to produce proteins that differ in their N-terminal domains (V-domains), but are the same elsewhere (C domains) (11-13). Ig V region domains from the heavy and light chain polypeptides (V_H and V_L) pair to form the ligand binding region (14). By analogy, it seems likely that the binding site for antigen and MHC is formed by pairs of TcR V-domains (either α:β or γ:δ). In the Ig variable regions, sequence diversity is concentrated in three distinct 'hypervariable regions'(15, 16). These amino acids form the principal points of contact with antigens and are thus referred to as complementarity determining regions (CDR's) (17, 18).

Sequence data suggest that TcR variable regions fold into a ß sheet tertiary structure similar to Ig variable regions (19-24). In antibodies, the variable regions from the heavy and light chains (V_H and V_L) are paired such that the three complementarity regions (CDR1, 2, and 3) from each domain form the antigen binding site (17, 18, 25). The overall geometry of V_L-V_H pairing is conserved in the Fab's whose structures are known (26, 27) resulting in a similar arrangement of CDR's in these binding sites. Most of the amino acids involved in the interface between Ig V_H and V_L are identically placed in TcR V region sequences (20-22, 24), suggesting that the overall geometry of the TcR V_α:V_β and V_γ:V_δ combining sites will be similar to that of V_H:V_L.

The three dimensional structures of a number of proteolytic fragments (Fab's) of antibodies complexed to antigens have been described (28-31). By contrast, the mode of association between TcR's and their more complex ligand (antigen/MHC) is not as well understood. Here we compare the patterns of diversity of Ig's and TcR's, and present a model for TcR interaction with a complex of MHC plus antigen. The model assumes structural similarity between the Ig and TcR combining sites in order to align the TcR V domains over the known structure of an MHC molecule (10, 32).

Table 1. Sequence Diversity in T Cell Receptor and Immunoglobulin Genes

	IG		TCR I		TCR II	
	H	κ	α	β	γ	δ
Variable segments	250-1000	250	100	25	7	10
Diversity segments	10	0	0	2	0	2*
D's read in all frames	rarely	-	-	often	-	often
N-region addition	V-D, D-J	None	V-J	V-D,D-J	V-J	V-D1,D1-D2, D1-J
Joining segments	4	4	50	12	2	2
Variable region combinations	62,500-250,000		2,500		70	
Junctional combinations	$\sim 10^{11}$		$\sim 10^{15}$		$\sim 10^{18}$	

Potential Diversity of TcR's Compared to Ig's

Compared to Ig's, the generation of diversity in TcR heterodimers indicates a striking concentration of sequence polymorphism in the CDR3-equivalent region (13). As indicated in Table I, there are significantly fewer TcR V gene segments than Ig V gene segments, and much less combinatorial diversity (V_H x V_κ vs. V_α x V_β, for example). By contrast, the diversity at the V-J junction of TcR's (CDR3) greatly exceeds that of Ig's. Particularly striking is the case of the adult TcRδ chain which seems to express only a few Vδ sequences but has been estimated to have up to 10^{13} possible amino acid sequences in its V-J region (33). The unique features of TcR genes that contribute to diversity in this region are listed in Table I and include N region addition in all four TcR chains (versus only V_H of immunoglobulins), the large number of J_α and J_β gene segments and the use of two different D regions simultaneously in TcR δ (13, 33, 34).

What this skewing of diversity towards the CDR3 equivalent region of TcR's might mean is suggested by the fact that in an antibody combining site, the CDR3 residues are located in the middle, in between the CDR1 and CDR2 contributed residues of each V region (25). In the HLA-A2 molecule, the putative peptide binding region is located in between two nearly parallel α helices on the surface of the structure. The distance between those two α-helices (~18 Angstroms) is almost identical to the distance between the CDR1 and CDR2 of one Ig V domain (in a heterodimer or homodimer) and another. Thus, an Ig molecule (or TcR) can be 'fit' over an MHC structure such that the CDR3 equivalent residues are spanning a significant portion of the apparent antigen binding site (13). This may explain the peculiar patterns of diversity that we see in TcR's versus Ig's and has interesting evolutionary predictions as well (see ref. 13).

ACKNOWLEDGMENTS

M.M.D. is a scholar of the PEW Memorial Trust, P.J.B. is a Postdoctoral Fellow of the American Cancer Society. We also wish to thank the NIH and the Howard Hughes Medical Institute for grant support.

REFERENCES

1. D. H. Katz, T. Hamaoka, and B. Benacerraf. Cell interactions between histoincompatible T and B lymphocytes. II. Failure of physiologic cooperative interactions between T and B lymphocytes from allogeneic donor strains in humoral response to hapten-protein conjugates. J. Exp. Med. 137:1405 (1973).
2. A. S. Rosenthal, and E. M. Shevach. Function of macrophages in antigen recognition by guinea pig T lymphocytes. J. Exp. Med. 138:1194 (1973).
3. R. M. Zinkernagel, and P. C. Doherty. Restriction of in vitro T-cell mediated cytotoxicity in lymphocytic choriomeningitis within a syngeneic or semi-allogeneic system. Nature 248:701 (1974).
4. B. Benacerraf. A hypothesis to relate the specificity of T lymphocytes and the activity of I region-specific Ir genes in macrophages and B lymphocytes. J. Immunol. 120:1809 (1978).
5. R. Shimonkevitz, J. W. Kappler, P. Marrack, and H. M. Grey. Antigen recognition by H-2 restricted T cells. I. Cell free antigen processing. J. Exp. Med. 158:303 (1983).
6. B. P. Babbitt, P. M. Allen, G. Matsueda, E. Haber, and E. R. Unanue. Binding of immunogenic peptides to Ia histocompatibility molecules. Nature 317:359 (1985).
7. S. Buus, S. Colon, C. Smith, J.H. Freed, C. Miles, and H. M. Grey. Interaction between a "processed" ovalbumin peptide and Ia molecules. Proc. Natl. Acad. Sci. USA 83:3968 (1986).
8. A. R. M. Townsend, J. Rothbard, G. M. Gotch, G. Bahadur, D. Wraith, and A. J. McMichael. The epitopes of influenza nucleoprotein recognized by cytotoxic T lymphocytes can be defined with short synthetic peptides. Cell 44:959 (1986).
9. J-G. Guillet, M-Z. Lai, T. J. Briner, J. A. Smith, and M. L. Gefter. Interaction of peptide antigens and class II major histocompatibility complex antigens. Nature 324:260 (1986).
10. P. J. Bjorkman, M. A. Saper, B. Samraoui, W. S. Bennett, J. L. Strominger, and D. C. Wiley. Structure of the human class I histocompatibility antigen, HLAL-A2. Nature 329:506 (1987).
11. S. Tonegawa. Somatic generation of antibody diversity. Nature 302:575 (1983).
12. M. Kronenberg, G. Sui, L. E. Hood, and N. Shastri. The molecular genetics of the T-cell antigen receptor and T-cell antigen recognition. Ann. Rev. Immunol. 4:529 (1986).
13. M. M. Davis, and P. J. Bjorkman. T cell antigen receptor genes and T cell recognition. Nature 334:395 (1988).
14. H. N. Eisen. "Immunology," Harper & Row, New York, (1980).
15. T. T. Wu, and E. A. Kabat. Analysis of the sequences of the variable regions of Bence-Jones proteins and myeloma light chains and their implications for antibody complementarity. J. Exp. Med. 132:211 (1970).
16. E. A. Kabat, T. T. Wu, M. Reid-Miller, H. M. Perry, and K. S. Gottesman. "Sequences of Proteins of Immunological Interest", Public Health Service, NIH, Bethesda, Maryland, 1987.
17. L. M. Amzel, and R. J. Poljak. Three-dimensional structure of immunoglobulins. Ann. Rev. Biochem. 48:961 (1979).
18. D. R. Davies, and H. Metzger. Structural basis of antibody function. Ann. Rev. Immunol. 1:87 (1983).
19. P. Patten, T. Yokota, J. Rothbard, Y. Chien, K. Arai, and M. M. Davis. Structure, expression and divergence of T cell receptor beta-chain variable regions. Nature 312:40 (1984).
20. R. Barth, B. Kim, N. Lan, T. Hunkapiller, N. Sobieck, A. Winoto, H. Gershenfeld, C. Okada, D. Hansburg, I. Weissman, and L. Hood. The murine T-cell receptor uses a limited repertoire of expressed V_b gene segments. Nature 316:517 (1985).
21. B. Arden, J. Klotz, G. Sui, and L. Hood. Diversity and structure of genes of the alpha family of mouse T-cell antigen receptor. Nature 316:783 (1985).

22. D. M. Becker, P. Patten, Y. Chien, T. Yokota, Z. Eshhar, M. Giedlin, N. R. J. Gascoigne, C. Goodnow, R. Wolf, K. Arai, and M. M. Davis. Variability and repertoire size in T cell receptor V and V_β gene segments. Nature 317:430 (1985).
23. S. M. Hedrick, E. A. Nielsen, J. Kavaler, D. I. Cohen, and M. M. Davis. Sequence relationships between putative T-cell receptor polypeptides and immunoglobulins. Nature 308:153 (1984).
24. J. Novotny, S. Tonegawa, H. Saito, D. M. Kranz, and H. N. Eisen. Secondary, tertiary, and quaternary structure of T-cell-specific immunoglobulin-like polypeptide chains. Proc. Natl. Acad. Sci. USA 83:742 (1986).
25. C. Chothia, and A. M. Lesk. Canonical structures for the hypervariable regions of immunoglobulins. J. Mol. Biol. 196:901 (1987).
26. J. Novotny, and E. Haber. Structural invariants of antigen binding: Comparisons of immunoglobulin V_L-V_H and V_L-V_L domain dimers. Proc. Natl. Acad. Sci. USA 82:4592 (1985).
27. C. Chothia, J. Novotny, R. Bruccoleri, and M. Karplus. Domain association in immunoglobulin molecules. The packing of variable domains. J. Mol. Biol. 186:651 (1985).
28. A. G. Amit, R. A. Mariuzza, S. E. V. Phillips, and R. J. Poljak. Three-dimensional structure of an antigen-antibody complex at 2.8 A resolution. Science 233:7474 (1986).
29. P. M. Colman, W. G. Laver, J. N. Varghese, A. T. Baker, P. A. Tulloch, G. M. Air, and R. G. Webster. Three-dimensional structure of a complex of antibody with influenza virus neuraminidase. Nature 326:358 (1987).
30. S. Sheriff, E. W. Silverton, E. A. Padlan, G. H. Cohen, S. J. Smith-Gill, B. C. Finzel, and D. R. Davies. Three-dimensional structure of an antibody-antigen complex. Proc. Natl. Acad. Sci. USA 84:8075 (1987).
31. D. M. Segal, E. A. Padlan, G. H. Cohen, S. Rudikoff, M. Potter, and D. R. Davies. The three-dimensional structure of a phyosphorylcholine-binding mouse immunoglobulin Fab and the nature of the antigen binding site. Proc. Natl. Acad. Sci. USA 71:4298 (1974).
32. P. J. Bjorkman, M. A. Saper, B. Samraoui, W. S. Bennett, J. L. Strominger, and D. C. Wiley. The foreign antigen binding site and T cell recognition regions of Class I histocompatibility antigens. Nature 329:512 (1987).
33. J. F. Elliott, E. P. Rock, P. A. Patten, M. M. Davis, and Y. Chien. The adult T-cell receptor δ-chain is diverse and distinct from that of fetal thymocytes. Nature 331:627 (1988).
34. Y. Chien, M. Iwashima, D. A. Wettstein, K. B. Kaplan, J. F. Elliott, W. Born, and M. M. Davis. T-cell receptor δ gene rearrangements in early thymocytes. Nature 330:722 (1987).

HUMAN T CELL RECEPTOR $\gamma\delta$ STRUCTURE

Michael B. Brenner[*^] Frans Hochstenbach[*], Hamid Band[*], Christina Parker[*], Joanne McLean[*], Shingo Hata[#], and Michael Krangel[#]

[*]Laboratory of Immunochemistry, Dana Farber Cancer Institute
[^]Department of Rheumatology and Immunology, Brigham and Women's Hospital
[#]Division of Tumor Virology, Dana Farber Cancer Institute
Harvard Medical School, Boston, MA., USA

A subpopulation of peripheral blood T-lymphocytes exists that is distinct from T cells that express the T cell receptor (TCR) $\alpha\beta$. This population of T cells expresses a receptor composed of TCR γ and TCR δ polypeptides that are associated with CD3 (Brenner et al., 1986). The TCR γ gene (Saito et al., 1984; Quertermous et al., 1986) has been extensively examined and is composed of variable (V), joining (J), and constant (C) region gene segments that undergo somatic rearrangement during development (Hayday et al., 1985).

TCR δ GENE

Recently, a gene has been cloned in mouse (Chien et al., 1987a) and man (Hata, Brenner, and Krangel 1987) that encodes the TCR δ subunit. To isolate the human gene, a T cell-specific cDNA probe was generated by synthesizing ^{32}P-labeled first strand cDNA of high specific activity from polyadenylated RNA of a TCR $\gamma\delta$ cell line, IDP2. After subtraction of this material by hybridization to B cell RNA, a λ gt10 cDNA library from the IDP2 cell line was probed. One group of cDNA clones (Group O) was characterized in detail because they detected cross-hybridizing mRNA from cell lines known to express the TCR $\gamma\delta$, but not from B cell or TCR $\alpha\beta^+$ T cells. In addition, the gene corresponding to these clones appeared to be deleted from T cells known to express the TCR $\alpha\beta$, and to undergo rearrangement in TCR $\gamma\delta$ lymphocytes when compared to non T cells. Deduced amino acid sequence analysis revealed that this gene encodes a V, J and C regions analogous to immunoglobulins and other T cell receptor genes. In particular, the V region (V δ1) is identical to V at 75% of selected consensus residues. Similarly the J region is highly homologous to Jα consensus residues as well as to Jβ and Jγ sequences. The C region displays low homology to Cα, Cβ and Cγ. It is composed of an immunoglobulin-like domain and a membrane spanning domain containing basic residues that are spaced similarly to those of the corresponding region in Cα. Recent studies indicate that while limited germline V-gene diversity exists for TCR δ, remarkable diversity exists in the region of the V-J junction (Hata et al., 1988). This region appears to be encoded by two tandemly arranged diversity (D) elements, with interspersed N segments (Chien et al. 1987b; Hata et al., 1988). The V-J junction thus provides TCR δ with unprecedented diversity localized predominantly at this location.

To confirm that the gene characterized above, in fact, encodes the TCR δ subunit, we demonstrated that it could be recognized by a specific monoclonal antibody (mAb). The mAb, anti-TCR δ 1, was made against TCR $\gamma\delta$ -CD3 protein that was isolated by co-immunoprecipitation from the PEER cell line using anti-CD3 mAb. MAb anti-TCR δ 1 binds to the surface of all TCR γδ cell lines thus far examined (>50 independently derived cell lines) and it immunoprecipitates the TCR γδ complex or the TCR δ chain alone (Band et al., 1987). One candidate TCR δ cDNA clone was placed in the pGEM3 expression vector. RNA transcripts were generated in the presence of T7 RNA polymerase. These transcripts were then placed in a rabbit reticulocyte lysate _in vitro_ translation reaction mixture in the presence of ^{35}S-methionine. Anti-TCR δ 1 directly recognized the polypeptide whose synthesis was directed by the TCR δ candidate cDNA clone, indicating that the cDNA clone, in fact, corresponds to the gene encoding the TCR δ subunit.

THREE TCR γδ FORMS

In man, the TCR γδ receptor complex is known to occur in both disulfide and nondisulfide-linked forms (Brenner et al. 1987). These forms correspond to usage of the Cγ1 or Cγ2 constant region gene segments, respectively (Littman et al. 1987; Krangel et al. 1987). The Cγ1 gene segment is encoded by three exons. The CI exon encodes an immunoglobulin-like constant domain, the CIII exon encodes the transmembrane region and the connecting piece between these two regions is encoded by the CII exon. The disulfide and the nondisulfide-linked forms are determined by the sequence of the respective CII exons. For Cγ1 genes, the CII exon encodes a cysteine residue that is implicated in interchain disulfide-linkage, while the CII exons of Cγ2 lack such a cysteine residue. The disulfide-linked (Cγ1) derived TCR γ chain is 40 kD while the nondisulfide-linked TCR γ chain was found in two cell surface polypeptide sizes, 55 kD or 40 kD (Brenner et al. 1987, Hochstenbach et al. 1988). The 55 kD nondisulfide-linked TCR γ chain is encoded by the Cγ2 gene that consists of three related CII exons, copies a, b, and c. Such multiple CII exon copies result in an extended connector region and encode 4 potential asparagine-linked oligosaccharide addition sites, all of which appear to be used. The additional polypeptide length and glycosylation result in a 55 kD cell surface TCR γ polypeptide chain. However, recently we have found a shorter nondisulfide-linked TCR γ polypeptide chain of 40 kD. Analysis of a cDNA clone encoding this form reveals use of the Cγ2 gene segment consisting of two rather than three CII exons, namely copies b and c. Interestingly, the absence of CII exon copy "a" (only 48 bp) results in a rather dramatic size difference in the cell surface TCR γ chain (40 versus 55 kD). This difference in size between these two nondisulfide-linked TCR γ chains is largely accounted for by the attachment of less N-linked carbohydrate in the shorter (40 kD) form. This appears to occur because of a change in conformation of the polypeptide chain that results from the absence of the CII exon copy "a". Thus unusual difference in glycosylation of two proteins that have the same number of potential N-linked glycan acceptor sites but very differently use such sites highlights the structural distinctness of these two nondisulfide-linked forms. The two nondisulfide-linked forms probably correspond to two genomic alleles of the Cγ2 gene (LeFranc et al. 1986; Pelicci et al. 1987). Based on Cγ gene and CII exon usage we refer to the three forms as Form 1 (disulfide-linked, Cγ1 encoded) and Form 2abc or Form 2bc (nondisulfide-linked, Cγ2 encoded) and consisting of three (copies a, b, and c) or two (copies b and c) of the CII exons, respectively.

These structurally distinct isotypic forms are not know to be functionally different, however, work in this area is currently under investigation. Now that the genes and the proteins that comprise the TCR γδ are known and mAb that allow the cells to be readily detected have been produced, it should be possible to define the role this subpopulation of T cells plays in the immune system.

REFERENCES:

1. Brenner, M.B., McLean, J., Dialynas, D.P., Strominger, J.L., Smith, J.A., Owen, F.L., Seidman, J.G., Ip, S., Rosen, F., and Krangel, M.S. Identification of a putative second T-cell receptor. Nature 322:145-149 (1986).

2. Brenner, M.B., McLean, J., Scheft, H., Riberdy, J., Ang, S.-L., Seidman, J.G., Devlin, P., and Krangel, M.S. Two forms of the T-cell receptor gamma protein found on peripheral blood cytotoxic T lymphocytes. Nature 325:689-694 (1987).
3. Chien, Y., Iwashima, M., Kaplan, K.B., Elliott, J.F., and Davis, M.M. A new T-cell receptor gene located within the alpha locus and expressed early in T-cell differentiation. Nature 327:677-682 (1987).
4. Chien, Y-h., Iwashima, M., Wettstein, D.A., Kaplan, K.B., Elliot, J.F., Born, W., Davis, M.M. T-cell receptor δ gene rearrangements in early thymocytes. Nature 330:722-727 (1987).
5. Hata, S., Brenner, M.B., and Krangel, M.S. Identification of putative human T cell receptor δ complementary DNA clones. Science 238:678-682 (1987).
6. Hata, S., Satyanarayana, K., Devlin, P., Band, H., McLean, J., Strominger, J.L., Brenner, M.B., Krangel, M.S. Extensive junctional diversity of rearranged human T cell receptor δ genes. Science 240:1541-1544 (1988).
7. Hayday, A.C., Saito, H., Gillies, S.D., Kranz, D.M., Tanigawa, G., Eisen, H.N., and Tonegawa, S. Structure, organization, and somatic rearrangement of T cell gamma genes. Cell 40:259-269 (1985).
8. Hochstenbach, F., Parker, C., McLean, J., Gieselmann, V., Band, H., Bank, I., Chess, L., Spits, H., Strominger, J.L., Seidman, J.G., Brenner, M.B. Characterization of a third form of the human T-cell receptor $\gamma\delta$. J Exp Med 168:761-776 (1988).
9. Krangel, M.S., Band, H., Hata, S., McLean, J., and Brenner, M.B. Structurally divergent human T cell receptor g proteins encoded by distinct $C\gamma$ genes. Science 237:64-67 (1987).
10. LeFranc, M.-P., Forster, A., and Rabbitts, T.H. Genetic polymorphism and exon changes of the constant regions of the human T-cell rearranging gene γ. Proc. Natl. Acad. Sci. USA 83:9596-9600 (1986b).
11. Littman, D.R., Newton, M., Crommie, D., Ang, S.-L., Seidman, J.G., Gettner, S.N., and Weiss, A. Characterization of an expressed CD3- associated Ti γ -chain reveals $C\gamma$ domain polymorphism. Nature 326:85-88 (1987).
12. Pelicci, P.G., Subar, M., Weiss, A., Dalla-Favera, R., and Littman, D.R. Molecular diversity of the human T-gamma constant region genes. Science 237:1051-1055 (1987).
13. Quertermous, T., Murre, C., Dialynas, D., Duby, A.D., Strominger, J.L., Waldman, T.A., and Seidman, J.G. Human T-cell γ chain genes: Organization, diversity, and rearrangement. Science 231:252-255 (1986).
14. Saito, H., Kranz, D.M., Takagaki, Y., Hayday, A.C., Eisen, H.N., and Tonegawa, S. Complete primary structure of a heterodimeric T-cell receptor deduced from cDNA sequences. Nature 309:757-762 (1984).

THE ROLE OF THE ZETA CHAIN IN THE EXPRESSION, STRUCTURE AND FUNCTION OF THE T CELL RECEPTOR

Richard D. Klausner, Allan M. Weissman, Michal Baniyash,
Juan S. Bonifacino and Lawrence E. Samelson

Cell Biology and Metabolism Branch, National Institute of Child
Health and Human Development, National Institutes of Health
Bethesda, MD

INTRODUCTION

The T Cell Antigen Receptor (TCR) is an extremely complex cell surface receptor that plays a key role in both the development and mature function of the immune system serving the dual functions of antigen recognition and transmembrane signaling[1,2]. The overall structure of the receptor and how it generates appropriate physiologic transmembrane signals is the object of studies in our laboatory. Two types of components make up the TCR: 1) clonotypic chains (Ti alpha and beta or Ti gamma and delta) provide the recognition function and antigen-MHC specificity of the receptor; and 2) non-polymorphic chains (CD3) most likely determine the signalling capacity of the receptor. The receptor is defined structurally by the non-covalent assemblage of a clonotypic heterodimer with the complete set of CD3 chains. This requisite co-assembly is underscored by the fact that the lack of any of the above components leads to a deficiency in the surface expression of the multichain complex. The most recently characterized component of the receptor complex is the zeta chain[3-5]. This was first observed in murine and subsequently found in human T cells. Zeta is a 16 kD protein as determined by migration on SDS-PAGE. It is found only in T cells and exists primarily as a homodimer. Its pI of 8.2-8.3 makes it the most basic of all of the components of the surface TCR and it carries no N-linked carbohydrate as determined by both metabolic labeling and treatment with endoglycosaminidases.

MOLECULAR CLONING OF THE ZETA cDNA

Purification of murine zeta chains allowed for the production of anti-zeta antibodies which recognize no other TCR components and, due to cross reaction, allowed for the initial identification of the human zeta. Further, purification of immunoprecipitated zeta on non-reducing/reducing PAGE gels allowed for protein sequencing of mature zeta to be carried out. Based on protein sequence, oligonucleotide probes were designed and used to isolate cDNA's encoding the murine zeta chain[6]. We have used the zeta cDNA to isolate the corresponding human cDNA and murine and human genes. The murine zeta chain is encoded by a single gene which produces a 1.7-1.8 kb message. This mRNA in only found in T cells. A 1.2 kb cDNA which encodes the zeta protein was sequenced. A single open reading frame predicts a 164 amino acid protein with a molecular wright of 18,637. Hydrophobicity analysis demonstrates an amino terminal hydrophobic region suggestive of a leader peptide and a single additional hydrophobic stretch compatable with a transmembrane helix[7]. Further analysis of the amino terminus by the method of von Heijne strongly points to this region being a leader peptide with the predicted site of cleavage between amino acids 21 and 22[8]. Such a cleavage would result in a mature protein whose 143 residues has a molecular weight of 16,299. A model of zeta reveals an unusual transmembrane protein. It contains only 9 extracellular amino acids followed by a 21 amino acid transmembrane segment. The carboxy terminal 113 amino acids form a long cytoplasmic tail. No nucleotide or amino acid sequence similarity was observed between zeta and any of the other components of the TCR or to any other known protein. One interesting feature is shared by zeta and all of the other TCR components. The predicted transmembrane region of zeta contains a single negative charge. All of the other CD3 components similarly possess a negatively charged residue in their predicted transmembrane domains[9-11]. The clonotypic components contain positively charged residues in these hydrophobic domains[12-14]. The presence of charges in these regions is a very unusual feature for transmembrane proteins. A single cysteine at the external face of the membrane spanning domain defines the site of disulfide bond formation. Finally six intracytoplasmic tyrosines are potential sites for the phosphorylation of zeta that is seen upon receptor activation. One additional feature of zeta revealed by the sequence is a possible binding site for ATP due to the presence of a consensus sequence (Gly-x-Gly-x-x-Gly-x-x-x-Gly...Ala-x-Lys) first recognized in protein kinases and which is found at the carboxy terminus of the zeta protein[15].

In vitro translation of RNA transcripts made from the cloned cDNA resulted in the production of an 18.5 kD protein that was immunoprecipitated by two different anti-zeta antisera. When translation was carried out in the presence of dog pancreas microsomes the 18.5 kD protein was largely processed to a 16 kD form consistent with SDS-PAGE migration of mature T cell zeta and again, was specifically recognized by anti-zeta antibodies. An antibody raised in rabbits against a peptide present in the predicted sequence, recognized zeta in murine T cells further confirming the identity of the clone. The murine cDNA clone was used to screen a human cDNA library derived from T cells. The human zeta clone recognized a 1.9 to 2.0 kb mRNA expressed only in T cells. Sequencing of the human cDNA showed a very high degree of conservation in the protein coding region (85% nucleotide, 87% amino acid). All of the following features are conserved between mouse and man: 1) the extracellular domain; 2) the single cysteine; 3) the intramembrane aspartate; 4) all intracellular tyrosines; and 5) the possible ATP binding consensus sequence. As would be expected, in contrast to the high degree of conservation in the protein sequence of the mature subunit, the leader sequence is only 50% conserved.

ROLE OF ZETA IN THE EXPRESSION OF THE TCR

In studies of the biosynthesis, assembly and fate of the components of the TCR in murine antigen specific T cell hybridomas, we noted that four of the chains of the TCR, alpha, beta, delta and epsilon were synthesized in great excess of the amount that survived to be expressed at the cell surface[16]. The excess proteins were (90%) transported from the site of synthesis in the ER through the Golgi where carbohydrate processing was completed only to be rapidly degraded, most likely by transport to lysosomes. Two other chains, CD3-gamma and zeta, were degraded to a much lesser extent. This was particularly true of zeta for which there was little rapid degradation following synthesis. These data, and other information, suggested that gamma and zeta were limiting for the assembly of complete receptor complexes in these cells and that only complete complexes were capable of avoiding this intracellular lysosomal degradation and be efficiently transported to and stably expressed on the cell surface. It was thus particularly interesting and particularly fortunate to be able to study the post-biosynthetic fate of the TCR in a variant of the 2B4 hybridoma which was isolated and cloned at the NIH by Jon Ashwell[17]. This variant, termed MA 5.8, made normal amounts of alpha, beta and CD3-gamma, -delta and -epsilon but made no detectable zeta chain by metabolic pulse labeling. Northern blot analysis of RNA derived from MA 5.8 failed to detect any zeta mRNA in these cells. Southern blotting with the murine zeta cDNA revealed identical restriction fragments in MA 5.8 and in the parent cell, 2B4. The assembly and carbohydrate processing of the TCR chains in these cells occurred with identical kinetics and to an identical extent to that seen in the parental cells.

However, whereas in the parental 2B4 cells the vast majority of the fully assembled "heptamer" (alpha, beta, gamma, delta, epsilon, $zeta_2$) was transported to the cell surface and survived for long periods of time only 3-5% of the assembled "pentamer" (alpha, beta, gamma, delta, epsilon) in the zeta-deficient cell survived rapid lysosomal degradation. This 3-5% was expressed on the cell surface and quantitative FACS analysis using either anti-alpha or anti-epsilon revealed that MA 5.8 expressed 3-5% as many receptors on the surface as the parental cell. The enhanced rapid degradation of newly synthesized chains seen in MA 5.8 could be blocked by drugs that inhibit lysosomal proteolysis. This lead us to conclude that zeta plays a unique role in preventing the sorting of incompletely assembled complexes to the lysosomes.

ROLE OF ZETA IN THE STRUCTURE OF THE TCR: INCREASING COMPLEXITY

In the TCR the vast majority of zeta exists as a disulfide-linked homodimer. When the TCR from murine T cells are examined after either extrinsic labeling or metabolic labeling by immunoprecipitation followed by resolution of the complex on two dimensional diagonal gels, two substoichiometric disulfide linked structures are observed below the diagonal in the same general areas where the zeta homodimer is seen. These spots migrate together in the non-reduced dimension at an apparent M_r of 38 kD which after reduction, resolve into proteins with apparent M_r's of 22 and 16 kD. After dissociation of the TCR complex the zeta homodimer and the p16-p22 heterodimer are still quantitatively precipitated by anti-zeta antibodies. When the p16 component of the heterodimer is subjected to proteolysis it yields a peptide map identical to zeta. In contrast when p22 is similarly analyzed its peptide map bears no resemblance to zeta or to any other component of the CD3 complex. Like zeta, p22 has no N-linked carbohydrate chains. Quantitation by a number of techniques all allowed us to conclude that, in 2B4 hybridoma cells, 10% of zeta is present as part of the heterodimer. What is particularly intriguing is the observation that in peripheral T cells (derived from spleen) and in a variety of T cell lines, hybridomas and tumors, very similar distribution of zeta between homodimer and heterodimer is seen. We have chosen to refer to the disulfide linked p22 as the eta chain of the TCR[18]. The fact that, even on cloned T cells, 10% of zeta exists linked to eta suggest that 20% of TCR complexes contain the zeta-eta dimer. This, in turn, suggests that there may be two classes of TCR molecules on the cell surface; 20% containing zeta-eta and 80% lacking zeta-eta. The functional significance of this is currently being evaluated.

THE ZETA CHAIN IS TYROSINE PHOSPHORYLATED UPON RECEPTOR ACTIVATION

Activation of the T cell via the TCR can be induced by multiple stimuli. These include antigen, mitogen, anti-receptor antibodies and certain antibodies directed against a variety of proteins on the T cell surface. The biochemical events that follow receptor stimualtion give us critical clues as to the processes of T cell activation. Proximal events in what are likely to be complex biochemical cascades include phosphoinositide metabolism and the stimulation of tyrosine phosphorylation events[19]. Several substrates within the cell are rapidly phosphorylated including a subunit of the receptor complex. This phosphoprotein migrated under reducing conditions with an M_r of 21 kD and we referred to this phosphorylated subunit as p21. The efficient precipitation of phospho-p21 by anti-zeta antibodies even under conditions that lead to subunit dissociation and in human cells in which zeta does not co-immunoprecipitate with the other receptor components suggested a close structural relationship between zeta and p21. Under non-reducing conditions phospho-p21 migrates with an M_r of 32 kD. Like both zeta and eta, phospho-p21 contains no N-linked carbohydrate chains. However, its migration fits with neither zeta nor eta on two dimensional non-reducing/reducing SDS-PAGE. No metabolically labeled protein co-migrates with phospho-p21 on these gels if cells are not activated. However, upon activation a previously metabolically labeled protein appears with these mobility characteristics. Alkaline phosphatase treatment of immunoprecipitates from such labeled activated cells results in the specific disappearance of this "spot". If this activation-related protein is isolated from the two dimensional gel and subjected to alkaline phosphatase treatment it can be identified as zeta by two criteria: 1) it now co-migrates with zeta on one dimensional reducing SDS-PAGE; and 2) it has an identical partial peptide map to zeta and is different than eta. Thus, zeta is the tyrosine phosphorylated TCR subunit. Even at maximum stimulation only 5-10% of zeta is tyrosine phosphorylated. Recent data suggests that multiple tyrosines on zeta are cooperatively phosphorylated during activation and that this is responsible for the dramatic mobility shift (both M_r and pI) of zeta after phosphorylation. The functional role of zeta phosphorylation in T cell activation remains to be determined.

The availability of zeta deficient cells which express pentameric receptor (alpha, beta, gamma, delta, epsilon) on their surface allowed us to evaluate the role of zeta in receptor mediated signal transduction[17]. Variant lines of the parental antigen-specific hybridoma were selected that matched the low number of surface TCR molecules found in the zeta negative cells but which contained all TCR components were used as controls. In the absence of zeta the cells were unable to respond to antigen or antibodies directed against Thy 1. This was measured as the absence of IL-2 production or phosphatidylinositol turnover. Interestingly these zeta negative receptors could be stimulated via direct cross linking of the CD3-epsilon chain using a monoclonal anti-epsilon antibody. Thus the zeta-negative receptors could not mediate signals stimulated by antigen or accessory molecules but could couple to biochemical activation pathways if directly cross linked. These results suggest a role for zeta in translating cell surface occupancy into transmembrane signalling.

REFERENCES

1. Marrack, P. & Kappler, J. (1986) Adv. Immunol. 38, 1-24.
2. Weiss, A., Imboden, J., Hardy, K., Manger, B., Terhorst, C. & Stobo, J. (1986) Ann. Rev. Immunol. 4, 593.
3. Samelson, L. E., Harford, J. B. & Klausner, R. D. (1985) Cell 43, 223-231.
4. Oettgen, H. C., Pettey, C. L., Maloy, W. L. & Terhorst, C. (1986) Nature (London) 320, 272-275.
5. Weissman, A. M., Samelson, L. E. & Klausner, R. D. (1986) Nature 324, 480-482.
6. Weissman, A. M., Baniyash, M., Hou, D., Samelson, L. E., Burgess, W. H. & Klausner, R. D. (1988) Science, in press.
7. Kyte, J. & Doolittle, R. (1982) J. Mol. Biol. 157, 105.
8. von Heijne, G. (1986) Nucl. Acids Res. 14, 4683.
9. Van den Elsen, P., Shepley, B. A., Borst, J., Coligan, J. E., Markham, A. F., Orkin, S. & Cox, C. (1984) Nature 312, 413-418.
10. Gold, D. P., Puck, J. M., Pettey, C. L., Cho, M., Coligan, J., Woody, J. N. & Terhorst, C. (1986) Nature 321, 431-434.
11. Krissansen, G. W., Owen, M. J., Verbi, W. & Crumpton, M. J. (1986) EMBO J. 5, 1799-1808.
12. Saito, H., Kranz, D. M., Takagaki, Y., Hayday, A. C., Eisen, H. N. & Tonegawa, S. (1984) Nature 309, 757-762.
13. Chien, Y-H., Iwashima, M., Kaplan, K. B., Elliot, J. F. & Davis, M. M. (1987) Nature 327, 677-682.
14. Brenner, M. B., Dialynas, D. P., Strominger, J. L., Smith, J. A., Owen, F. L., Seidman, J. G., Ip, S., Rosen, F. & Krangel, M. S. (1986) Nature 302, 145-149.
15. Kampo, M. P. et al. (1984) Nature 310, 589.
16. Minami, Y., Weissman, A. M., Samelson, L. E. & Klausner, R. D. (1987) Proc. Natl. Acad. Sci. USA 84, 2688.
17. Sussman, J. J., Baonifacino, J. S., Lippincott-Schwartz, J., Sato, T., Klausner, R. D. & Ashwell, J. (1988) Cell 52, 85.
18. Baniyash, M., Garcia-Morales, P., Bonifacino, J., Samelson, L. E. & Klausner, R. D. (1988) J. Biol. Chem., 263, 9874-9878.
19. Patel, M. D., Samelson, L. E. & Klausner, R. D. (1987) J. Biol. Chem. 262, 5831-5838.

USE OF SOMATIC CELL MUTANTS TO STUDY THE SIGNAL TRANSDUCTION FUNCTION OF THE T CELL ANTIGEN RECEPTOR

Mark A. Goldsmith, Linda K. Bockenstedt, Paul Dazin and Arthur Weiss

Departments of Medicine and of Microbiology and Immunology
Howard Hughes Medical Institute
University of California, San Francisco
San Francisco, CA

INTRODUCTION

The activation of thymus-derived lymphocytes (T cells) is regulated by cell surface molecules that may function in a stimulatory or inhibitory manner. Among the many plasma membrane proteins that have been implicated in T cell functional activities, the antigen receptor plays a central role in initiating T cell activation during an immune response. Upon appropriate interaction with antigen or anti-receptor antibodies that have been used to mimic antigen, the T cell receptor induces transmembrane signalling events that contribute to the subsequent cellular response. Such cellular activation is most commonly manifested by the appearance of cytolytic activity, production of lymphokines or proliferation of T cells.

The T cell antigen receptor on most human T cells is a multi-chain molecular complex consisting of a disulide-linked α/β heterodimer (Ti) associated with the 5-7 invariant chains comprising the CD3 complex.[1,2] A distinct heterodimer, the Tiγ/δ receptor, is associated with CD3 on a small number of T cells that lack CD4 and CD8 antigens, as well as Ti α/β heterodimers. Whereas all four of the Ti chains are derived from rearranging immunoglobulin-like genes, the genes of the CD3 chains that have been identified do not undergo rearrangements. CD3 and Ti are intimately associated on unstimulated cells[3-6] and this association is obligatory for cell surface expression of the CD3 complex.[7] The structural basis for this association is as yet undefined.

The Ti α/β subunit functions in the recognition of both nominal antigen and the restricting major histocompatibility molecule.[8,9] However, due to the relatively short cytoplasmic domains of the α and β chains, the signal transducing function of the receptor is thought to be performed by the associated invariant CD3 complex. The notion that CD3 may play a role in signal transduction is supported primarily by the demonstration that anti-CD3 monoclonal antibodies can function as agonists, thereby mimicking the effects of antigen.[2]

Transmembrane signalling by the CD3/Ti complex has been studied in considerable detail. Antigen, agonist CD3 or Ti mAb, or T cell mitogenic lectins that depend upon CD3/Ti expression all initiate a common transmembrane signal by inducing the hydrolysis of phosphatidylinositol 4,5-bisphosphate (PIP_2).[2,10] This results in the generation of two potent second messengers, inositol 1,4,5-trisphosphate (IP_3) and diacylglycerol (DAG), which in turn induce an increase in cytoplasmic free calcium

($[Ca^{2+}]_i$) and activation of protein kinase C (pkC), respectively.[11]
Both the increase in $[Ca^{2+}]_i$ and activation of pkC have been implicated indirectly in many of the cellular responses of T cell activation. How perturbation of the CD3/Ti complex results in the hydrolysis of PIP_2 is as yet unclear, but this process may depend upon guanyl nucleotide-binding proteins that could serve to couple CD3/Ti to an intracellular phospholipase C.[12]

In an effort to relate the structure of the CD3/Ti complex to its signal transducing function, we have begun to derive somatic cell signalling mutants of the T cell line Jurkat.[13] This approach circumvents the difficulties in studying a receptor composed of such a large number (7-9) polypeptide chains. Here, we describe the partial characterization of one of these mutants and relate its signalling defects to cellular responses. In addition we have utilized this signalling mutant as well as receptor-loss mutants to study the relative role of the antigen receptor in signal transduction by the CD2 molecule, another cell surface receptor that can mediate transmembrane signalling events similar to those of the CD3/Ti complex.

RESULTS AND DISCUSSION

The derivation of the signalling mutant J.CaM1

The human T cell leukemic line Jurkat has been utilized by our laboratory for the characterization of transmembrane signalling events mediated by the antigen receptor.[2] Jurkat expresses a CD3-associated Ti α/β heterodimer that is recognized by the clonotypic monoclonal antibody (mAb) C305.[14] C305 or anti-CD3 mAb induce the hydrolysis of PIP_2 and increase $[Ca^{2+}]_i$ in Jurkat cells.[2]
Likewise, in a CD3/Ti-dependent manner, the lectins concanavalin A (Con A) and phytohemagglutinin (PHA) mediate similar transmembrane signalling events. In a previous report, we described a selection protocol for the isolation of mutants of Jurkat with defective CD3/Ti transmembrane signalling function and presented the preliminary characterization of one such mutant.[13] The isolation of such mutants relies on a multistep selection protocol (summarized in Figure 1). A key to this protocol was the observation that PHA inhibits the growth of Jurkat cells in a CD3/Ti-dependent fashion. This PHA-mediated growth inhibition is likely to be the consequence of transmembrane signalling events initiated through CD3/Ti. After several weeks in culture, PHA-resistant cells could be isolated from an initial culture of mutagenized Jurkat cells. A substantial proportion of these cells failed to express the receptor; an anticipated class of signalling mutant would be represented by a receptor-loss phenotype. However, of greater interest are those cells that continue to express cell surface CD3/Ti since it is among these cells that mutants in the proximal components of

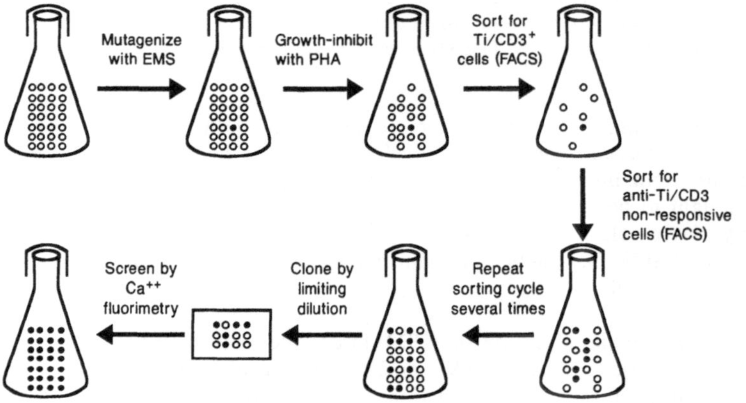

Figure 1. Derivation of a T cell antigen receptor (CD3/Ti) signalling mutant.

Table 1. A Proximal Defect in Transmembrane Signalling Events in J.CaM1.

	Jurkat			J.CaM1		
	Basal	OKT3	C305	Basal	OKT3	C305
$[Ca^{2+}]_i$*	87	976	1923	92	70	62
Inositol Phosphates**						
IP_3	100	355	397	100	110	126
IP_1+IP_2	100	502	616	100	104	97
Phosphatidic Acid***	100	374	409	100	91	97

*Basal or peak cytoplasmic free calcium ($[Ca^{2+}]_i$); nM.
**Inositol trisphosphate (IP_3), inositol monophosphate (IP_1), inositol bisphosphate (IP_2); percent of basal levels after ten minutes of stimulation.
***Phosphatidic acid, percent of basal levels after ten minutes of stimulation.

the signal transduction apparatus should be found. Following the enrichment of CD3/Ti-bearing cells on a fluorescence activated cell sorter (FACS), we utilized the FACS and the calcium-sensitive fluorescent dye Indo-1[15] to enrich for cells that failed to increase $[Ca^{2+}]_i$ in response to C305. The cell sorting enrichment procedures were repeated several times in order to isolate a large population of receptor-bearing C305-unresponsive cells, which were then cloned by limiting dilution. The first such signalling mutant, J.CaM1, is described in further detail.

Characterization of the J.CaM1 signalling phenotype

In our initial evaluation of J.CaM1, we examined the ability of these cells and the wildtype Jurkat cells to respond to anti-CD3 (OKT3) and anti-Ti (C305) mAb. We first compared the ability of these agonists to induce increases in $[Ca^{2+}]_i$ in the two cells. In contrast to the substantial increases $[Ca^{2+}]_i$ observed in Jurkat cells, no increases are observed in J.CaM1 cells to either of these agonist mAb (Table 1). Since the increase in $[Ca^{2+}]_i$ is thought to be a consequence of PIP_2-derived inositol phosphates, we examined the ability of C305 and OKT3 to induce PIP_2 hydrolysis in J.CaM1. Neither of these mAb produce an increase in either the phosphatidylinositol-derived inositol phosphates or the DAG metabolite, phosphatidic acid (Table I). These results suggest that the defect in J.CaM1 involves a relatively proximal component of the transmembrane signalling apparatus since increases in early second messengers derived from PIP_2 hydrolysis are undetectable.

We then extended our analysis to a larger panel of agonists in an effort to gain some insight into the defect in J.CaM1. J.CaM1 is unresponsive to any of three available anti-Ti mAb that function as agonists in Jurkat cells (Table 2), despite the ability of all three of these mAb to recognize antigenic determinants expressed on J.CaM1 at levels comparable to or slightly greater than those on Jurkat cells (not shown). Likewise, some anti-CD3 (OKT3, UCHT1, A32.1) fail to induce increases in $[Ca^{2+}]_i$, yet others (Leu 4, 235, L142) do induce substantial increases in $[Ca^{2+}]_i$ (Table 2).

The ability of anti-CD3 mAb to function as agonists does not correlate with their reactivity with J.CaM1 since all of the CD3 antibodies bind to J.CaM1 to a comparable

Table 2. Lack of Responsiveness of J.CaM1 is Only Partial.

Stimulus	Specificity	Isotype	Responding cell Jurkat	J.CaM1
C305	Ti	IgM	1923*	82
R140	Ti	IgG	650	73
WT31	Ti	IgG	567	106
OKT3	CD3	IgG	976	70
Leu 4	CD3	IgG	1322	243
UCHT1	CD3	IgG	336	80
235	CD3	IgM	831	710
L142	CD3	IgM	1634	971
A32.1	CD3	IgG	1117	86

* Peak increase in $[Ca^{2+}]_i$, nM.

extent. Although the most potent anti-CD3 agonists for J.CaM1 are of the IgM isotype, we do not believe this reflects their ability to cross-link the receptor since C305, the anti-Ti used in selecting the unresponsive phenotype, is also a decavalent IgM mAb. Interestingly, combinations of some non-agonist anti-Ti and anti-CD3 mAb can induce substantial increases in $[Ca^{2+}]_i$.[13] This is observed even with an Fab fragment of one anti-CD3 used with intact anti-Ti. Thus, these findings suggest that the transmembrane signalling function of the CD3/Ti complex is only partially defective in J.CaM1 and that appropriate perturbation of the complex may be able to initiate transmembrane signalling events.

Collectively, these observations would suggest that the defect in J.CaM1 is not in a distal component of the signalling pathway since, with appropriate stimuli, hydrolysis of PIP_2 (not shown) and increases in $[Ca^{2+}]_i$ can be induced. More importantly, these studies are most consistent with a model of the CD3/Ti complex in which conformational changes within the receptor complex are responsible for the initiation of the signal transduction pathway. Hence, the defect in J.CaM1 may lie in a region involving the association between Ti and CD3, resulting in the inability of all anti-Ti and only some anti-CD3 mAb to induce the appropriate conformational change in the CD3/Ti complex. In support of this model in which the CD3/Ti complex represents a conformationally-dependent receptor are previous studies in which certain, but not all, anti-Ti mAb reactive with the cell line HPB-ALL can function as agonists in signal transduction.[16]

Localizing the defect in J.CaM1

We have begun to localize the defect in J.CaM1 through a complementation analysis. Since the Ti α and ß chains are allelically excluded, they are effectively haploid genes. Therefore, we have initially focused our attention on these molecules as only a single mutation would be required to alter the function of either of these chains; this model would also be consistent with the inability of all anti-Ti mAb examined to function as agonists in J.CaM1. As an initial approach, stable somatic cell hybrids have been prepared between J.CaM1 and mutants of the Jurkat line that fail to express functional α or ß chain transcripts, and as a result lack the CD3/Ti complex on the plasma membrane. Both of these deficient mutants could complement J.CaM1 as demonstrated by the ability of the hybrid cells to respond to C305.[17] Since analysis of stable hybrids has some ambiguity due to the potential complementation of defects in the parental lines (i.e., complementation by J.CaM1 of α or ß chain transcription in the expression mutant fusion partners) we have developed another method for the complementation of J.CaM1.[18]

This method involves examining the signalling capability of heterokaryons formed from J.CaM1 and a variety of other cells that lack or ß chain transcripts. Such an analysis can be performed within 15 minutes after fusion and avoids the possible induction or extinction of gene expression in stable hybrids. Preliminary results from this analysis have also excluded the Ti α or ß chains as being the site of the defect in J.CaM1. These surprising results suggest that the defect in J.CaM1 may reside in a CD3 chain or closely associated structure. Importantly, these results would also support a model in which Ti is unable to initiate transmembrane signalling alone, but requires the participation of another functionally-linked structure, i.e., CD3.

<u>Altered cellular responses to defective transmembrane signalling in J.CaM1</u>

A number of cellular responses have been related to transmembrane signalling events initiated by the CD3/Ti complex. For instance, an increase in $[Ca^{2+}]_i$ and the activation of pkC have been causally implicated in the events leading to the transcriptional activation of the interleukin 2 (IL-2) gene.[2] In support of this, in contrast to the ability of OKT3 or C305 plus phorbol myristate acetate (PMA) to induce IL-2 production by Jurkat, J.CaM1 fails to produce IL-2 in response to either of these combinations of stimuli.[13] The defective receptor in J.CaM1 can be bypassed through the use of a calcium ionophore and PMA, which together induce IL-2 production in Jurkat and J.CaM1.[13] These results lend support to the importance of the CD3/Ti-mediated PIP_2 hydrolysis with consequent $[Ca^{2+}]_i$ increase and pkC activation in the events leading to IL-2 gene activation, although we cannot exclude the possibility that another signal transduction system mediated by CD3/Ti is also defective in J.CaM1.

In light of the ability of mAb 235 to increase $[Ca^{2+}]_i$ in J.CaM1, if the increase in $[Ca^{2+}]_i$ and activation of pkC are causally related to IL-2 production, 235 plus PMA would be expected to activate J.CaM1 to produce IL-2. Surprisingly, J.CaM1 fails to produce detectable IL-2 or its transcripts in response to 235 plus PMA.[19] This observation challenged the notion that the increase in $[Ca^{2+}]_i$ and activation of pkC are necessary for IL-2 production. However, analysis of the inositol phosphates generated in response to 235 reveals a striking difference between J.CaM1 and Jurkat. The peak inositol phosphate response is markedly attenuated in J.CaM1, and IP_3 and its metabolites return to basal levels more rapidly. Likewise, in a reexamination of the increase in $[Ca^{2+}]_i$ in J.CaM1, we found that although the increase over the first 20 minutes is comparable to that seen in Jurkat, $[Ca^{2+}]_i$ returns to basal levels at 60 to 90 minutes.[19] These results are compatible with the notion that the failure of J.CaM1 to produce IL-2 in response to 235 and PMA may reflect the transient nature of the increase in $[Ca^{2+}]_i$ induced by 235. These results are also consistent with previous studies that demonstrated that persistant CD3/Ti-dependent signalling for 4 hours is necessary for Jurkat commitment to IL-2 secretion.[20] These studies strongly argue that early receptor-mediated signal transduction events must be interpreted with caution, as they may be insufficient to induce cellular responses unless they are sustained.

Another response to mAb that bind to the receptor involves the internalization of both CD3 and Ti components of the complex (also referred to as modulation).[21] Several investigators have demonstrated that PMA can also induce a down-regulation of CD3/Ti expression and have indirectly linked the concomitant phosphorylation ofCD3γ and δ chains to receptor internalization.[22,23] Since anti-Ti and anti-CD3 mAb induce pkC activation as a result of PIP_2 hydrolysis and also induce phosphorylation of CD3γ and δ chains, it has been speculated that antibody-induced internalization of CD3/Ti is a consequence of pkC-mediated phosphorylation of the CD3 chains. Since no demonstrable PIP_2 hydrolysis occurs following the binding of C305 to the receptor on J.CaM1 cells, we could test the relationship of the transmembrane signalling events to CD3/Ti internalization. Indeed, CD3 and Ti determinants are modulated to a comparable extent on both J.CaM1 and Jurkat cells that have been incubated with C305 mAb.[13] This result would suggest that mAb-induced receptor modulation is independent of transmembrane signalling events and, presumably, CD3γ and δ chain phosphorylation.

Table 3. CD2-Mediated Increases in $[Ca^{2+}]_u$ Depend Upon the Expression of a Functional CD3/Ti Complex.

Responding cell	Phenotype	Basal	Anti-CD2*
Jurkat	wildtype	91	356
J.RT3-T3.5	Ti ß-, CD3/Ti-	59	76
PF-2.4	Ti ß transfectant, CD3/Ti+	67	530
J.CaM1	signalling mutant	90	90

*Peak $[Ca^{2+}]_i$ (nM) following the addition of anti-CD2 mAb 9.6+9.1.

Expression and normal function of the CD3/Ti complex is required for transmembrane signalling via the CD2 complex. CD2 is a single chain 50 kD cell surface protein expressed on T cells, NK cells and thymocytes.[1] CD2 can be stimulated by appropriate combinations of mAb to induce a variety of the manifestations of T cell activation including IL-2 production, proliferation and induction of cytolytic activity. Recently, lymphocyte function antigen-3 (LFA-3), a 55-70 kD glycoprotein expressed on a wide variety of hematopoietic cells has been shown to be a physiologic ligand of CD2.[24] As CD2 is a nonpolymorphic receptor and does not interact directly with antigen, activation of cells via CD2 has been termed an alternative pathway of activation. Interestingly, transmembrane signalling via CD2 also involves the phosphatidylinositol pathway.[25] Thus, two receptors with very distinct structural features and ligands, CD2 and the CD3/Ti complex, mediate similar signal transduction events.

Several recent studies have suggested that the CD3/Ti complex and CD2 may functionally interact. A dependence upon CD3/Ti expression has been demonstrated in some cells stimulated with agonist combinations of CD2 mAb,[26,27] although this is not uniformly observed. In addition, synergistic effects upon cellular responses have been observed when CD3/Ti and CD2 are simultaneously stimulated with combinations of mAb.[28] Therefore, we examined the ability of activating combinations of CD2 ligands to initiate transmembrane signalling events in 1) Jurkat; 2) J.RT3-T3.5, a mutant of Jurkat that fails to express ß chain transcripts resulting in the absence of cell surface CD3/Ti; 3) PF-2.4, a cell derived from J.RT3-T3.5 in which a ß chain cDNA has been expressed, resulting in reconstitution of cell surface CD3/Ti; and 4) J.CaM1, the signalling mutant described above. We found that the activating combination of anti-CD2 mAb 9.6 and 9-1 could initiate signal transduction in wildtype Jurkat cells but in neither the antigen receptor-negative mutant J.RT3-T3.5 nor in the signalling mutant J.CaM1 (Table 3). Signal transduction was restored in the ß chain reconstituted cell, PF-2.4, derived from the CD3/Ti negative mutant. In preliminary studies, similar observations were made in this panel of cells when the natural ligand LFA-3 was used under appropriate conditions.[27] Collectively, these results indicate that at least in Jurkat cells, signal transduction by CD2 is dependent not only on expression of a CD3/Ti complex, but also upon its function. The mechanism underlying this dependence is as yet unclear.

CONCLUSIONS

The T cell antigen receptor is a complex structure comprised of 7-9 chains that functions in antigen recognition and in signal transduction. To analyze how the structure of the receptor relates to its signal transducing function, we have begun to derive somatic cell mutants with defective signalling function using a generalizable protocol. We have also begun the initial characterization of one such mutant, J.CaM1. J.CaM1 appears to contain a defect within the proximal components of the signal transduction, perhaps within the CD3/Ti complex itself. A prelimary complementation analysis has ruled out the α and ß chains as the site of the defect, making it tempting to speculate that the defect may lie within CD3 or a closely associated structure. From the analysis of J.CaM1, we conclude that the CD3/Ti complex is dependent upon conformational changes to initiate transmembrane signalling events and that Ti alone does not contain sufficient information for the initiation of signal transduction. We suggest that the stimulation of Ti by antigen results in a conformational change in Ti which is perceived by the CD3 complex, and then amplified into a signal that can effectively activate coupling and effector mechanisms involved in signal transduction.

Using J.CaM1, we examined the relationship of several cellular responses to signal transduction events mediated by CD3/Ti. These studies of J.CaM1 have reinforced the notion that an increase in $[Ca^{2+}]_i$ and activation of pKC are important events that contribute to the activation of the IL-2 gene. It appears likely that such transmembrane signals must be persistant in order to result in the transcriptional activation of the IL-2 gene. Hence, transmembrane signals may not always lead to a cellular response. How such transmembrane signals contribute to the transcriptional activation of the IL-2 gene is as yet undefined. Additionally, since we found that the CD3/Ti complex on J.CaM1 is internalized in response to anti-Ti mAb in the absence of detectable PIP_2 hydrolysis, it would seem that at least one form of CD3/Ti internalization is independent of CD3 phosphorylation.

At least one other receptor on human T cells, CD2, mediates signal transduction events similar to those of the CD3/Ti complex. The striking difference in the structure of these receptors, as well as previous observations suggesting their possible functional interaction, led us to examine the dependence of CD2 upon CD3/Ti. These studies clearly demonstrated that, at least on Jurkat, signal transduction competence of CD2 is dependent upon the expression and normal function of the CD3/Ti complex. The basis of this functional dependence remains to be explored.

The complexity of the T cell antigen receptor has hampered the study of how it participates in initiating T cell activation. The derivation of a large panel of somatic cell signalling mutants should provide a useful approach towards the study of structural and functional relationships among various components of the T cell antigen receptor and other cellular components involved in the signal transduction apparatus. Moreover, it should provide useful model systems for receptor reconstitution studies and for testing how some of the cellular responses are linked to receptor-mediated transmembrane signalling events.

ACKNOWLEDGEMENTS

The authors would like to thank Michael Armanini for his help in the preparation of this manuscript. M.A.G. is supported by the Rosalind Russell Arthritis Foundation and by the N.I.H. Medical Scientist Training Program. L.K.B. is the recipient of a Postdoctoral Training Award from the Arthritis Foundation. A.W. is an Assistant Investigator of the Howard Hughes Medical Institute and the recipient of an Arthritis Investigator Award.

REFERENCES

1. J. P. Allison, and L. L. Lanier, Structure, function and serology of the T-cell antigen receptor complex, Ann. Rev. Immunol. 5:503 (1987).
2. A. Weiss, J. Imboden, K. Hardy, B. Manger, C. Terhorst, and J. Stobo, The role of the T3/antigen receptor complex in T-cell activation, Ann. Rev. Immunol. 4:593 (1986).

3. J. Borst, S. Alexander, J. Elder, and C. Terhorst, The T3 complex on human T lymphocytes involves four structurally distinct glycoproteins, J. Biol. Chem. 258:5135 (1983).
4. E. L. Reinherz, S. C. Meuer, K. A. Fitzgerald, R. Hussey, J. Hodgdon, O. Acuto, and S. Schlossman, Comparison of T3-associated 49- and 43-kilodalton cell surface molecules on individual human T-cell clones: Evidence for peptide variability in T-cell structures, Proc. Natl. Acad. Sci. USA 80:4104 (1983).
5. J. P. Allison, and L. L. Lanier, Identification of antigen receptor-associated structures on murine T cells, Nature 314:107 (1985).
6. M. B. Brenner, I. S. Trowbridge, and J. L. Strominger, Cross-linking of human T cell receptor proteins: Association between the T cell idiotype beta subunit and the T3 glycoprotein heavy subunit, Cell 40:183 (1985).
7. P. S. Ohashi, T. W. Mak, P. Van den Elsen, Y. Yanagi, Y. Yoshikai, A. Calman, C. Terhorst, J. D. Stobo, and A. Weiss, Reconstitution of an active surface T3/T-cell receptor by DNA transfer, Nature 316:606 (1985).
8. Z. Dembic, W. Haas, S. Weiss, J. McCubrey, H. Kiefer, H. von Boehmer, and M. Steinmetz, Transfer of specificity by murine alpha and beta T-cell receptor genes, Nature 320:232 (1986).
9. T. Saito, A. Weiss, J. Miller, M. A. Norcross, and R. N. Germain, Specific antigen-Ia activation of transfected human T cells expressing murine Ti alpha/beta human T3 receptor complexes, Nature 325:125 (1987).
10. J. B. Imboden, and J. D. Stobo, Transmembrane signalling by the T cell antigen receptor, J. Exp. Med. 161:446 (1985).
11. M. J. Berridge, and R. F. Irvine, Inositol triphosphate, a novel second messenger in cellular signal transduction, Nature 312:315 (1984).
12. J. B. Imboden, D. M. Shoback, G. Pattison, and J. D. Stobo, Cholera toxin inhibits the T-cell antigen receptor-mediated increases in inositol triphosphate and cytoplasmic free calcium, Proc. Natl. Acad. Sci. USA 83:5673 (1986).
13. M. A. Goldsmith, and A. Weiss, Isolation and characterization of a T cell somatic mutant with altered signal transduction by the antigen receptor, Proc. Natl. Acad. Sci. USA 84:6879 (1987).
14. A. Weiss, and J. D. Stobo, Requirement for the coexpression of T3 and the T cell antigen receptor on a malignant human T cell line, J. Exp. Med. 160:1284 (1984).
15. G. Grynkiewicz, M. Poenie, and R. Y. Tsien, A new generation of Ca^{2+} indicators with greatly improved fluorescence properties, J. Biol. Chem. 260:3440 (1985).
16. L. L. Lanier, J. J. Ruitenberg, J. P. Allison, and A. Weiss, Distinct epitopes on the T cell antigen receptor of HPB-ALL tumor cells identified by monoclonal antibodies, J. Immunol. 137:2286 (1986).
17. M. A. Goldsmith, and A. Weiss, Generation and analysis of a T lymphocyte somatic mutant for studying molecular aspects of signal transduction by the antigen receptor. Ann. NY Acad. In press.
18. M. A. Goldsmith, P. F. Dazin, and A. Weiss, At least two non-antigen-binding molecules are required for signal transduction by the T cell antigen receptor, Proc. Natl. Acad. Sci. USA. In press.
19. M. A. Goldsmith, and A. Weiss, Early signal transduction by the antigen receptor without commitment to T cell activation, Science 240:1029 (1988).
20. A. Weiss, R. Shields, M. Newton, B. Manger, and J. Imboden, Ligand receptor interactions required for commitment to the activation of the interleukin 2 gene, J. Immunol. 138:2169 (1987).
21. S. C. Meuer, K. A. Fitzgerald, R. E. Hussey, J. Hodgdon, S. Schlossman, and E. Reinherz, Clonotypic structures involved in antigen-specific human T cell function. Relationship to the T3 molecular complex, J. Exp. Med. 157:705 (1983).
22. D. A. Cantrell, A. A. Davies, and M. J. Crumpton, Activators of protein kinase C down regulate and phosphorylate the T3/T-cell antigen receptor of human T lymphocytes, Proc. Natl. Acad. Sci. USA 82:8158 (1985).
23. L. E. Samelson, J. Harford, R. H. Schwartz, and R. D. Klausner, A 20-kDa protein associated with the murine T-cell antigen receptor is phosphorylated in response to activation by antigen or concanavalin A, Proc. Natl. Acad. Sci. USA 82:1969 (1985).

24. M. L. Plunkett, M. E. Sanders, M. Dustin, and T. A. Springer, Rosetting of activated T lymphocytes with autologous erythrocytes: Definition of the receptor and ligand molecules as CD2 and lymphocyte function-associated antigen-3 (LFA-3), J. Exp. Med. 165:664 (1987).
25. G. Pantaleo, D. Olive, A. Poggi, W. J. Kozumbo, L. Moretta, and A. Moretta, Transmembrane signalling via the T11-dependent pathway of human T cell activation. Evidence for the involvement of 1,2-diacylglycerol and inositol phosphates, Eur. J. Immunol. 17:55 (1987).
26. J. B. Breitmeyer, J. F. Daley, H. B. Levine, and S. F. Schlossman, The T11 (CD2) molecule is functionally linked to the T3/Ti T cell receptor in the majority of T cells, J. Immunol. 139:2899 (1987).
27. L. B. Bockenstedt, M. A. Goldsmith, M. Dustin, D. Olive, T. A. Springer, and A. Weiss, The CD2 ligand LFA-3 activates T cells but depends on the expression and function of the antigen receptor, J. Immunol. 141:1904 (1988).
28. S. Y. Yang, S. Chovaib, and B. Dupont, A common pathway for T lymphocyte activation involving both the CD3-Ti complex and CD2 sheep erythrocyte receptor determinants, J. Immunol. 137:1097 (1986).

CHANGES IN EARLY AND LATE STEPS OF T CELL ACTIVATION BY WT31 MoAb

Sudhir Gupta, Makito Shimizu, Renu Batra and Bharathi Vayuvegula

Division of Basic and Clinical Immunology, University of California, Irvine California, 92717

INTRODUCTION

The induction of T cell activation is usually a consequence of interaction between specific T cell receptors and their ligands. The T cell antigen receptor (TcR) is present on almost all T cells as a heterodimer of α and β glycoprotein (reviewed in 1). The TcR heterodimer is non-covalently associated with CD3 glycoprotein forming a TcR/CD3 complex (1). The TcR is responsible for antigen recognition and the CD3 antigen for signal transduction (reviewed in 2). Recently a monoclonal antibody (MoAb), WT31, has been described that recognizes a framework determinant present on all mature T lymphocytes that express α/β TcR heterodimer (3). In this investigation we have examined the effect of WT31 MoAb on some of the early and late steps of T cell activation to determine whether the WT31 moAb will induce signal transduction and activate human T cells. We show that WT31 activates human T cells via a classical signal transduction pathway.

MATERIALS AND METHODS

Peripheral venous blood was obtained from healthy adult donors. IL 2-dependent CTLL line is a gift from Dr. Steven Gillis, Immunex Corp., Seattle, WA. Purified WT31 moAb was a gift from Dr. Noel Warner, Becton-Dickinson, Mountain View, CA. Quin-2 AM dye was purchased from Molecular Probe, Junction City, OR. Recombinant IL-2 was purchased from AMGEN, Thousand Oaks, CA, and recombinant IL-1 from Genzyme, Cambridge, MA. Ion channel blockers 4 aminopyridine (4 AP), tetraethyleammonium (TEA), verapamil (Ver) and quinine (Q), and phorbol myristate acetate (PMA) were purchased from SIGMA, St. Louis, MO.

Isolation of Mononuclear Cells and Purification of T cells

Peripheral blood mononuclear cells were isolated on Ficoll-Hypaque density gradient. Cells were washed three times with Hanks' balanced salt solution (HBSS) and resuspended in medium-1640 (Irvine Scientific, Santa Ana, CA), supplemented with 100 U/ml penicillin, 100 ug/ml streptomycin, 2mM L-glutamine, 25 mM HEPES and 10% heat-inactivated fetal calf serum, hereafter referred to as culture medium (CM). T cells were purified by first removing adherent cells on Sephadex G-10 column followed by separation by nylon wool column. Cells eluted from the column were washed three times with HBSS and resuspended in CM at a desired concentration. T cells obtained were >98% pure as defined with anti-CD2 moAb using FACS.

Intracellular Calcium Measurements

Ten million cells in 1 ml of medium were loaded with 80 uM Quin 2 for 45 minutes at 37°C, washed x 2 with HBSS and then resuspended in saline solution containing (in mM) 145 NaCl, 1 Na_2HPO_4, 0.5 $MgSO_4$, 5 KCl, 1 $CaCl_2$, 5 glucose, and 10 HEPES (pH 7.4). Five million cells in saline solution were placed in a temperature controlled (37°C) quartz cuvette for each experiment, and measurements made with a Spectrofluorimeter (SPEX, Fluorog, Metuchen, NJ), with excitation at 339 nm and emission at 484 nm. Spectrofluorimeter output is recorded on FM tape and is digitized off line with a LSI-11/23 computer and data interface.

Measurement of Cell Volume

Mononuclear cells (3 x 10^6/ml) were stimulated with WT31, PMA or togethers for 48 hours at 37°C for 48 hours. Cells were washed three times with PBS and volumes were recorded using FACS. Gates were also set to determine the proportion of cells showing change in cell volume. The data are presented as mean log channels numbers.

Interleukin 2 (IL-2) Production

Peripheral blood mononuclear cells (2 X 10^6/ml) were incubated with WT31 moAb for 48 hours, supernatants collected, filtered and stored at -20°C until used. Unstimulated cell supernatants served as negative or background controls. Interleukin 2 activity was measured on IL 2-dependent CTLL cell line.

DNA Synthesis

One hundred microliters of peripheral blood mononuclear cells (MNC) in CM (1 x 10^6/ml) were dispensed in 96 round bottom well microtiter plates and stimulated with specified concentrations of WT31 moAb in the presence or absence of phorbol myristate acetate (PMA) or IL1 and/or IL-2 for specified time periods. The cultures were pulsed with 1 uCi/well of ^{3}H thymidine (New England Nuclear, Boston, MA.) for the final 18 hours of culture and ^{3}H thymidine incorporation was measured by scintillation counter. All experiments were done in triplicate and data are expressed as counts per minute (cpm; mean ± sd).

RESULTS

Concentration and Time-Kinetic of WT31-Induced Activation of T Lymphocytes

Mononuclear cells or purified T cells were stimulated with various concentrations of WT31 moAb for 3 days at 37° and cultures were pulsed with ^{3}H thymidine for an additional 18 hours. The results of ^{3}H thymidine incorporation are shown in Figure 1. Approximately 50-100 ng/ml of WT31 inducedd maximum DNA synthesis. Therefore, we used 100 ng/ml WT31 moAb to study the time-kinetic of DNA synthesis. Mononuclear cells or purified T cells were stimulated with WT31 moAb for one to 6 days at 37°C and DNA synthesis was measured. The results (Figure 2) show that the peak response for DNA synthesis was at 90 hours (3 days + 18 hours following addition of ^{3}H thymidine). It should be noted that the DNA synthesis was macrophage-dependent but purified T cell responses also peaked at day 3.

Effect of WT31 on Changes in Lymphocyte Volume

Mononuclear cells were stimulated with WT31, PMA, and WT31 plus PMA for 24 hours and volume changes were measured by FACScan. Figure 3 shows increased cell volume upon stimulation with WT31 and PMA. A further increase in cell volume was observed when lymphocytes were stimulated with WT31 plus PMA.

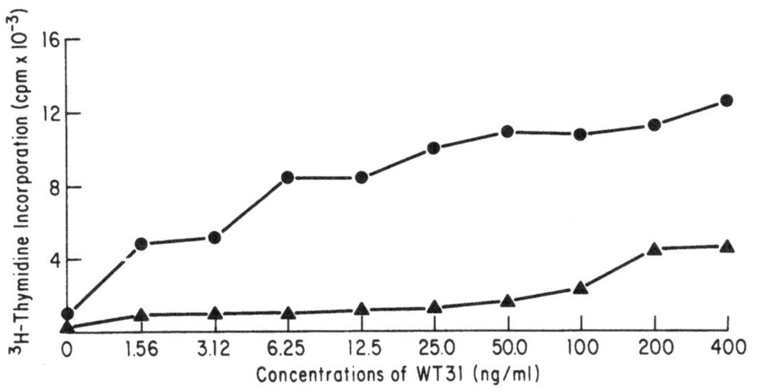

Figure 1. DNA synthesis with various concentrations of WT31 in the presence (●) or absence (▲) of monocytes.

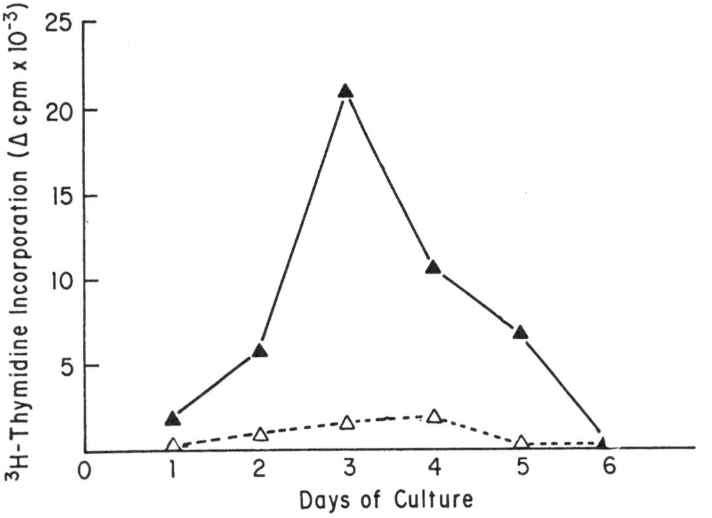

Figure 2. Time kinetics of WT31-induced (100 ng/ml) DNA synthesis in T cells.

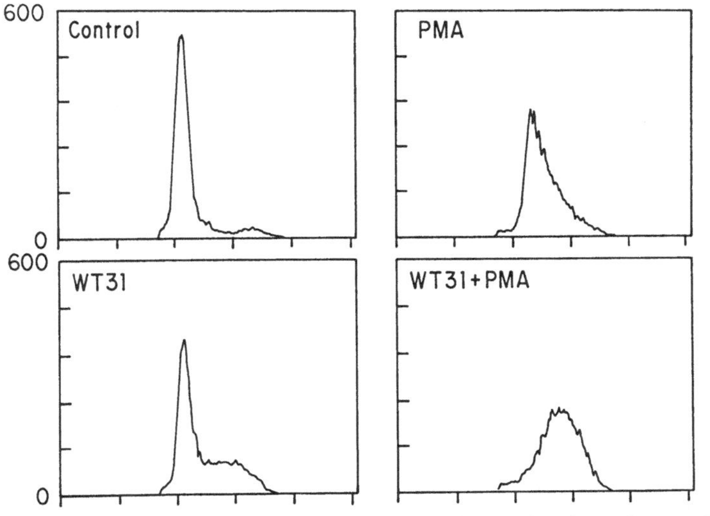

Figure 3. Changes in cell volume folowing activation with WT31.

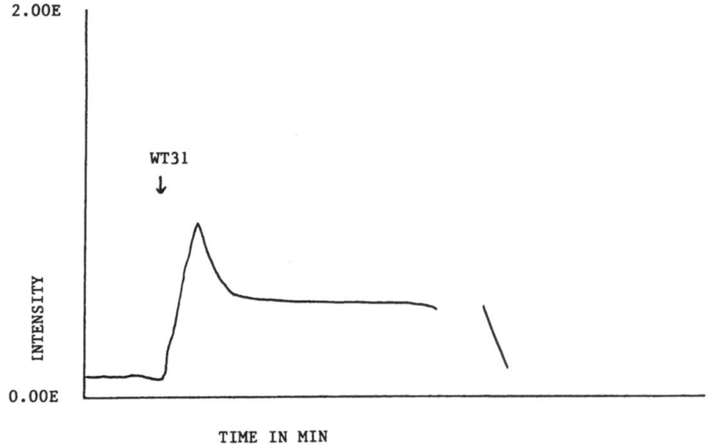

Figure 4. Changes in $[Ca^{++}]_i$ following activation with WT31.

Effect of WT31 on Intracellular Free Calcium $[Ca^{++}]_i$

Mononuclear cells were loaded with Quin 2 and intracellular calcium was measured with spectrofluorimeter. An increase in $[Ca^{++}]_i$ was observed following stimulation with WT31 (Figure 4).

WT31-Induced Interleukin 2 Production

Mononuclear cells were stimulated with various concentrations of WT31 for 24 hours and supernatants were collected and assayed for IL-2 activity on IL-2-dependent CTLL cell line. Recombinant IL-2 (rIL-2) was used as positive control. Activation of mononuclear cells resulted in IL-2 production (Table 1). Furthermore, a synergism was observed between WT31 and phorbol myristate acetate (PMA), a protein kinase C activator.

Table 1. Production of IL-2 by WT31-Stimulated Mononuclear Cells.

Exp. Conditions	^{3}H Thymidine Incorporation (cpm ± sd)
Cells alone	925 ± 229
rIL-2 (10 U/ml)	24,654 ± 2,966
rIL-2 (1 U/ml)	3,683 ± 326
WT31 (50 ng/ml)	4,090 ± 353
PMA (10 ng/ml)	9,806 ± 620
WT31 + PMA	22,356 ± 1,628

Mononuclear cells were stimulated with WT31, PMA or together for 48 hours. Supernatants were collected, filtered and assayed for IL-2 activity on a IL-2-dependent CTLL cell line against known concentrations of recombinant IL-2. Data are expressed as mean ± sd of 3 separate experiments.

Table 2. Effect of IL-1, IL-2 and Both on WT31-Activated Mononuclear Cells.

Cells	WT31	IL-1	IL-2	^{3}H thymidine Incorp. (cpm)
+	-	-	-	3,554 ± 1,106
+	50.0	-	-	17,740 ± 1,612
+	50.0	+	-	14,310 ± 1,228
+	50.0	-	+	27,601 ± 3,465
+	50.0	+	+	18,629 ± 1,191
+	25.0	-	-	16,751 ± 4,868
+	25.0	+	-	15,711 ± 2,201
+	25.0	-	+	28,650 ± 1,714
+	25.0	+	+	25,401 ± 2,913
+	12.5	-	-	11,752 ± 4,662
+	12.5	+	-	13,168 ± 863
+	12.5	-	+	23,886 ± 9,646
+	12.5	+	+	9,343 ± 784

Data are expressed as Mean ± SD of 3 separate experiments.

Recombinant Interleukin 2 Increases WT31-Induced DNA Synthesis

Mononuclear cells were stimulated with various concentrations of WT31 in the presence or absence of IL-1, IL-2, or both. Data in Table 2 show that recombinant IL-1 neither had any effect on WT31-induced DNA synthesis nor increased IL-2 enhanced DNA synthesis by WT31-activated mononuclear cells. Interleukin 2, as expected had an enhancing effect on WT31-induced DNA synthesis.

Effect Of Ion Channel Blockers on WT31-Induced DNA Synthesis

Mononuclear cells were stimulated with 50 ng/ml of WT31 in the presence or absence of various concentrations of K^+ channel blockers (4 AP, TEA), Ca^{++} channel blocker (Ver), and Ca^+-activated K^+ channel blocker (Q) for 3 days and ^{3}H thymidine incorporation was measured. The data in Table 3 show that all channel blockers in a dose-dependent manner inhibited DNA synthesis, suggesting a role of ion channels in WT31-induced DNA synthesis.

DISCUSSION

In this investigation we show that WT31 MoAb, which recognizes a framework determinants of α/β TcR gene products present on almost all peripheral blood T cells, activates T lymphocytes by a classical ligand-mediated signal transduction pathway.

WT31-induced DNA synthesis was monocyte-dependent (Figure 1). It appears that WT31 MoAb binds to Fc receptors of monocytes and therefore monocytes provide a matrix for cross-linking of WT31. Anti-CD3 monoclonal antibodies and clonotypic antibodies for TcR have also shown to to be monocyte-dependent for DNA synthesis and IL-2 production by T cells or T cell lines (4, 5). Anti-CD3 monoclonal antibody (6, 7) as well as monoclonal antibodies against CD2 (8, 9), CD5 (10) and CD28 antigen (11, 12), induces a rise in $[Ca^{++}]_i$. Activation of human T cells with WT31 also resulted in an increase in free $[Ca^{++}]_i$. The increase in $[Ca^{++}]_i$ was due to the mobilization of intracellular pool of Ca^{++} (initial rapid rise) as well as due to an influx of extracellular Ca^{++} (later sustained rise of $[Ca^{++}]_i$). The latter rise was markedly inhibited by EGTA

Table 3. Effect of Channel Blockers on WT31-Activated Mononuclear Cells.

TEA (mM)	4 AP(mM)	Quinine (uM)	Verapamil (uM)	^{3}H Thymidine Incorp. (cpm)
-	-	-	-	20,783 ± 1,437
0.125	-	-	-	20,409 ± 2,614
0.25	-	-	-	18,937 ± 1,500
0.50	-	-	-	17,190 ± 1,257
1.0	-	-	-	15,314 ± 405
2.0	-	-	-	12,116 ± 1,873
4.0	-	-	-	10,722 ± 2,468
8.0	-	-	-	9,781 ± 1,991
-	0.125	-	-	17,746 ± 1,845
-	0.25	-	-	16,575 ± 556
-	0.50	-	-	14,145 ± 1,399
-	1.0	-	-	8,678 ± 584
-	2.0	-	-	2,488 ± 263
-	4.0	-	-	1,486 ± 528
-	8.0	-	-	200 ± 65
-	-	1.25	-	21,096 ± 2,596
-	-	2.50	-	20,435 ± 2,725
-	-	5.0	-	16,425 ± 1,280
-	-	10.0	-	13,353 ± 1,789
-	-	20.0	-	11,904 ± 6,284
-	-	40.0	-	8,509 ± 1,339
-	-	80.0	-	4,246 ± 1,694
-	-	-	0.625	16,719 ± 893
-	-	-	1.25	17,811 ± 1,576
-	-	-	2.5	13,714 ± 1,503
-	-	-	5.0	11,636 ± 707
-	-	-	10.0	7,820 ± 1,304
-	-	-	20.0	3,672 ± 256
-	-	-	40.0	1,200 ± 223

Mononuclear cells were stimulated with WT31 (50 ng/ml) in the presence of absence of various concentrations of ion channel blockers for 3 days and ^{3}H thymidine incorporation was measured. Data are expressed as mean ± sd of 3 separate experiments. Viability of cells as determined by trypan blue dye exlusion was comparable in all samples.

(data not shown). Anti-CD3 also induces rise in $[Ca^{++}]_i$ by a similar mechanism (13). The role of extracellular calcium in WT31-induced T cell activation is further supported by the fact that EGTA in a dose-dependent fashion inhibits WT31-induced DNA synthesis and IL-2R expression (14).

The activation of lymphocytes with antigens and plant lectins is associated with increase in cell size. We also show that the activation of T cells with WT31 results in an increase in cell size. Meuer et al (15), using a clonotypic MoAb and T cell clones, show that the antigen-induced proliferation of T cells is mediated through an autocrine pathway involving endogenous IL-2 production, release, and subsequent binding to IL-2R. We show that WT31 MoAb induces IL-2 production in human T cells. Furthermore, we have also shown that WT31 induces the expression of IL-2R and that T cells respond to IL-2 by increasing DNA synthesis (14). During an activation of T cells, the first signal is provided by an antigen in contex with major histocompatibility class II and the second signal is produced by interleukin 1 (IL-1). In the present study we did not find any enhancing effect of IL-1 on WT31 induced DNA synthesis or DNA synthesis induced by WT31 and IL-2 together.

Membrane ion channels have been shown to play an important role in human T cell functions (16). We (17, 18) and others (19) have shown the presence of voltage-gated K^{++} channels in human T lymphocytes. Furthermore, we have reported that, in addition to K^+ channel blockers, calcium channel blockers as well as calcium-activated K^+ channel blockers will block the K^+ channel currents and will inhibit DNA and protein synthesis (20, 21). More recently, Kuno et al (22) have demonstrated the presence of a voltage- insensitive Ca^{++} channels in human helper T cell clones. In the present study we show that K^+, Ca^{++} and Ca^{++}-activated K^+ channel blockers inhibited WT31-induced DNA synthesis by peripheral blood T cells. This would suggest a role of ion channels in WT31-induced DNA synthesis. Recently it has been reported that G proteins modulate membrane ion channels. Interestingly, WT31 also activates humna T cells via activation of G protein (14).

In summary, WT31 MoAb, which defines a framework determinant of α/β TcR, activates T cells by a classical transduction mechanism.

ACKNOWLEDGEMENTS:

This work was supported by USPHS grants AI-26456 and GM-41514

REFERENCES

1. Meuer S., Acuto O., Hercend T., Schlossman S. and Reinherz E. The human T-cell receptor. Ann. Rev. Immunol. 2: 23, 1984
2. Weiss A., Imboden J., Hardy K., Manger B., Terhorst C., and Stobo J. The role of T3/antigen receptor complex in T cell activation. Ann. Rev. Immunol. 4: 593, 1986.
3. Spitz H., Borst J., Tax W., Capel P.J.A., Terhorst C., and de Vries D.E. Characterstics of a monoclonal antibody (WT31) that recognizes a common epitope on the human T cell receptor for antigen. *J. Immunol.* 135:1922-1928, 1985.
4. Smith K.G.C., Austyn J.M., Hariri G., Beverley P.C.L. and Morris P.J. T cell activation by anti-T3 antibodies: Comparision of IgG1 and IgG2b switch variants and direct evidence of accessory function of macrophage Fc receptors. *Eur. J. Immunol.* 16:478-486, 1986.
5. Rinnooy Kan E.A., Platzer E., Welte K., and Wang C.Y. Modulation induction of the T3 antigen by OKT3 antibody is monocyte-dependent. *J. Immunol.* 133:2979-2985, 1984.
6. Imboden J.B., Stobo J.D. Transmembrane signalling by the T cell antigen receptor. Perturbation of the T3-antigen receptor complex generates inositol phosphates and releases calcium ions from intracellular stores. *J. Exp. Med.* 161:446-456, 1985.
7. Imboden J., Weiss A., and Stobo J. The antigen receptor on a human T cell line initiates activation by increasing cytoplasmic free calcium. *J. Immunol.* 134:663-665, 1985.
8. Weiss M.J., Daley J.F., Hodgdon J.C., and Reinherz E.L. Calcium dependency of antigen-specific (T3-Ti) and alternative (T11) pathways of human T-cell activation. *Proc. Natl. Acad. Sci. (USA)* 81:6836-6340, 1984.
9. Breitmeyer J.B., Daley J.F., Levine H.B., and Schlossman S. F. The T11 (CD2) molecule is functionally linked to the T3/Ti T cell receptor in the majority of T cells. *J. Immunol.* 139:2899, 1987.

10. June C.H., Rabinowitch P.S., Ledbetter J.A. CD5 antibodies increase intracellular ionized calcium concentration in T cells. *J. Immunol.* 138:3299-3305, 1986.
11. Panteleo G.,OliveD., Harris D., Poggi A., Moretta L., and Moretta A. Signal transducing mechanisms involved in human T cell activation via surface T44 molecules. Comparison with signal transduced with the T cell receptor complex. *Eur. J. Immunol.* 16:1639, 1986.
12. Hara T., Fu S.M., and Hansen J.A. Human T cell activation. A new activation pathway used by a major T cell population via disulfide-bonded dimer of a 44 kilodalton polypeptide (9.3 antigen). *J. Exp. Med.* 161:1513-1624, 1985.
13. Weiss A., Imboden J. Shobach D., and Stobo J. Role of T3 surface molecules in the activation of human T cells: T3-dependent activation results in an increase in cytoplasmic free calcium. *Proc. Natl. Acad. Sci. (USA)* 81:4169-4173, 1984.
14. Gupta S., Shimizu M. and Vayuvegula B. T cell activation by antibody (WT31) recognizing α/β TcR. (Submitted).
15. Meuer S.D., Hussey R.E., Cantrell D.A., Hodgdon J.C., Schlossman S.F., Smith K.A., and Reinherz E.L. Triggering of the T3-Ti antigen receptor complex results in T cell clonal proliferation through an interleukin 2-dependent autocrine pathway. *Proc. Natl. Acad. Sci. (USA)* 81:1719, 1984.
16. Chandy K.G., DeCoursey T.E., Cahalan M.D., and Gupta S. Electroimmunology: The physiological role of ion channel in the immune system. *J. Immunol.* 135:787s-791s, 1985.
17. DeCoursey T.E., Chandy K.G., Gupta S. and Cahalan M.D. Voltage-gated K channels in human Tlymphocytes. A role in mitogenesis. *Nature* 307:465-471, 1984.
18. Cahalan M.D., Chandy K.G., DeCoursey T.E., and Gupta S. A voltage-gated K+ channel in human T lymphocytes. *J. Physiol.* 358: 468-471, 1985.
19. Matteson D.R. and Deutsch C. K^+ channels in T lymphocytes. A patch clamp study using monoclonal antibody adhesion. *Nature* 307:468-471, 1984.
20. Chandy D.G., DeCoursey T.E., Cahalan M.D., McLaughlin C. and Gupta S. Voltage-gated potassium channels are required for human T lymphocyte activation. *J. Exp. Med.* 160:369-385, 1985.
21. Gupta S. Autologous mixed lymphocyte reaction in man. XVII. In vitro effect of ion channel blocking agents on the autologous mixed lymphocyte reaction. *Cell. Immunol.* 104:290-295, 1987.
22. Kuno M., Gronzy J., Weyand C.M. and Gardner P. Single channel and whole cell recordings of mitogen-regulated inward currents in human cloned helper T lymphocytes. *Nature* 323:269-273, 1986.

INTERLEUKIN 1 AND INTERLEUKIN 2 RECEPTORS

INTERLEUKIN-1 INDUCED T-LYMPHOCYTE PROLIFERATION AND ITS RELATION TO IL-1 RECEPTORS

Charles A. Dinarello, Scott F. Orencole and Nerina Savage

Department of Medicine, Tufts University School of Medicine and New England Medical Center Hospital, Boston, MA 02111 and Department of Medical Biochemistry, Medical School, University of the Witwatersrand Johannesburg, South Africa

INTRODUCTION

Interleukin-1 (IL-1) is a polypeptide cytokine which possesses several biological properties including lymphocyte activation, fever, endothelial cell stimulation and mesenchymal tissue remodeling (reviewed in 1). In lymphocytes, fibroblasts, endothelial cells, and macrophages, IL-1 induces a variety of immunomodulatory molecules, such as more IL-2, granulocyte-macrophage colony stimulating factor, IL-6, and IL-1 itself.[2] Many of the biological properties of IL-1 are also observed with another polypeptide cytokine, tumor necrosis factor (TNF)[3]; however, IL-1 and TNF have distinct primary structures and cell receptors. IL-1 receptors are most numerous on fibroblasts[4] and T-cell lines.[5-7] These include the EL4 murine thymoma and LBRM line. The IL-1 cell surface binding protein (receptor) recognizes both beta and alpha forms of IL-1 has been demonstrated on several lymphocyte-derived cell lines as well as mature, circulating blood T-cells.[8]

The characteristic biological effect of IL-1 on T-lymphocytes has been well-described; IL-1 augments the proliferative response to sub-optimal concentrations of mitogens and antigens.[9-11] IL-1's effect on lymphocytes is often described as a "helper" factor; in this regard, IL-1 effects on T-lymphocyte activation are also observed employing agents that directly activate protein kinase C or increase cytosolic calcium.[12] In order for T-cells to pnrogress from a resting to a proliferative phase, interleukin-2 (IL-2) and expression of IL-2 receptors are required. IL-1 stimulates IL-2 production[13] and IL-2 receptor expression[6,14]; however, these T-cell responses to IL-1 are greatly increased (10-100-fold) when IL-1 is combined with mitogens, antigens, phorbol esters, or calcium ionophores.

The original D10.G4.1 murine cell line was described as an antigen specific T-helper line which proliferated to IL-1 in the presence of sub-optimal concentrations of a monoclonal antibody to the antigen receptor or to mitogens, similar to the response of thymocytes and other lymphocytes. However, the D10.G4.1 cells proliferated to IL-1 plus mitogens without a demonstrable increased production of IL-2.[15] Although these cells proliferate to exogenously added IL-2, the effect of IL-1 on these cells is attributed to IL-1-induced IL-2 receptors. Recent studies also suggest that D10.G4.1 cells, in the presence of IL-1 and the monoclonal antibody (anti-CD3) specific for the antigen receptor on these cells, induces IL-4 and that IL-1 and IL-4 act together to induce proliferation.[16,17] In addition to IL-4, mitogen-stimulated D10.G4.1 cells produce another growth factor, identified as granulocyte-macrophage colony stimulating factor (GM-CSF).[18] In these latter two studies, IL-1, in the absence of mitogen or anti-CD3, did not lead to proliferation.

In the present study, we describe a subclone of the D10.G4.1 cell line which proliferates to subfemtomolar concentrations of recombinant human IL-1 (beta or alpha) in the absence of mitogen or antigen. We describe in this paper the specific biological characteristics of these T-cells; in the accompanying study, we demonstrate how the specific proliferative responses are related to unique receptors for IL-1. These data suggest that IL-1 is direct growth factor for these cells.

We conclude that 1) IL-1 is a direct growth factor for these cells at attmolar concentrations, 2) proliferation correlates directly to presence of IL-1 in the culture, 3) anti-IL-1 but not anti-IL-2 or anti-IL4 blocks the proliferative response, and 4) there is a direct relationship of the magnitude of proliferation to IL-1 and either the number IL-1 receptors or affinity of IL-1 to specifically bind to these cells.

MATERIALS AND METHODS

Cell Lines

The original D10.G4.1 cell line was kindly provided by Dr. Charles Janeway (Yale University, New Haven, CT) and was maintained by weekly splitting employing irradiated (2500 rads) AKR/J mouse spleen cells (Jackson Laboratories, Bar Harbor, ME), rat spleen cell conditioned medium and the specific antigen for those cells, conalbumin (Sigma, St. Louis, MO). In a typical tritiated thymidine uptake assay, these cells proliferated to IL-1 in the presence of a sub-optimal concentration (1 ug/ml) phytohemagglutinin-P (PHA, Burroughs Wellcome, Research Triangle, NC) but, as reported in several studies, IL-1 has no effect on the proliferation of these cells in the absence of mitogen. In order to preserve these cells, aliquots were periodically frozen in 5% DMSO (Fisher) 95% fetal calf serum (FCS, Hyclone, Logan, UT) and stored at -70C. To test the survivability of these cells, aliquots were thawed and grown for several weeks. Some of these frozen-thawed aliquots were tested for responses to IL-1 and results indicated that some aliquots were more sensitive to IL-1 without PHA than in the presence of PHA. The D10.G4.1 subclone was selected for ultra sensitivity to IL-1 inducible proliferation after long-term incubation (12-18 days) post passage without the addition of any mitogen. Once selected, these cells were maintained in a similar fashion to the parent clone, by passage approximately every 7 days (when the cells density reached $2\text{-}5 \times 10^5$5 cells/ml). Passage of the cells consisted of a 1:6 dilution into fresh RPMI media containing 0.01M HEPES (Microbiological Associates, Walkerville, MD), 10% FCS and $1\text{-}3 \times 10^5$ gamma-irradiated AKR/J mouse splenocytes, conalbumin (100 ug/ml), and 5-10% rat conditioned medium. Bioassays were performed on cells 5-8 days post passage. The clone was designated D10S and was shown not to be infected with Mycoplasma organisms as determined by the Mycotrim Test, Hana, Inc., Berkeley, CA.

Anti-Sera

The specificities and neutralizing abilities of polyclonal rabbit anti-rhuIL-1b and anti-rhuIL-1a and have been previously described.[3,19] Anti-human recombinant IL-2 was purchased from Genzyme, Inc., Boston, MA. Anti-mouse IL-4, a monoclonal antibody used previously,[17,20] was kindly provided by Dr. William Paul, NIH, Bethesda, MD.

Bioassay

Bioassays with the D10S cells (1×10^5 cells/ml) or CTLL (4×10^5 cells/ml) were performed in triplicate in 96-well polystyrene flat bottom microtiter plates at volumes of 200 ul/well and incubated for 72 hours at 37C in 5% CO2. Biological activity was determined by DNA incorporation of ^{3}H-thymidine (New England Nuclear, Boston, MA, 1 uCi/well) added to all cultures 18 hours preharvest. The cultures were harvested by aspiration in water and the cellular debris was filtered through glass-fiber paper. The filter paper was cut and beta-radioactivity was counted in 2.5 ml of scintillation cocktail (Beckman).

RESULTS

Sensitivity of D10S Cells to Recombinant IL-1

The proliferative responses of D10S cells to IL-1 in the absence of mitogen have been consistently observed in the subfemtomolar range in over 100 assays. Nine assays distributed over the past two years were randomly selected for statistical analysis. As shown in Figure 1, half-maximal responses to rhuIL-1-b were observed at 400 fg/ml in the absence of mitogen. However, significant ($p<0.001$, Student's T-test) proliferation was also observed at 1000-10,000-fold lower concentrations of IL-1 (0.4 and 0.04 fg/ml). Even at 0..004 fg/ml ($4x10^{-18}$M), the proliferative response was significantly ($p<0.01$) greater than that for cells incubated without IL-1. Similar results were also observed for the rhu or murine IL-1α (data not shown). On the other hand, the presence of PHA reduces the proliferative response to IL-1 and this observation distinguishes the D10S subclone from the parent clone[15,16] and D10.G4.1 cells recently reported.[17,18] In contrast, the parent clone responses to IL-1 are greatly augmented by PHA. Half-maximal responses in the parent clone was observed at 500 pg/ml only in the presence of PHA whereas rhu IL-1ß alone had no effect (compare 80,000 to 800 cpm at 1 pg/ml).

Using direct counting of D10S cells, we observed a steady increase in the number of cells following splitting and antigen challenge until day 7, at which time the rate of growth began to slow (data not shown). At that time, the cells became increasingly sensitive to the growth promoting effect of IL-1. Accordingly, we tested the sensitivity of D10S cells on the 6th and 15th day following the splitting and re-feeding. The sensitivity of D10S cells to IL-1 is clearly greater on day 15 than day 6 after the antigen challenge. At $1x10^5$ cells/ml (the standard concentration used in these experiments), 0.4 fg/ml yielded a stimulation index of 6 over control (no IL-1) and this

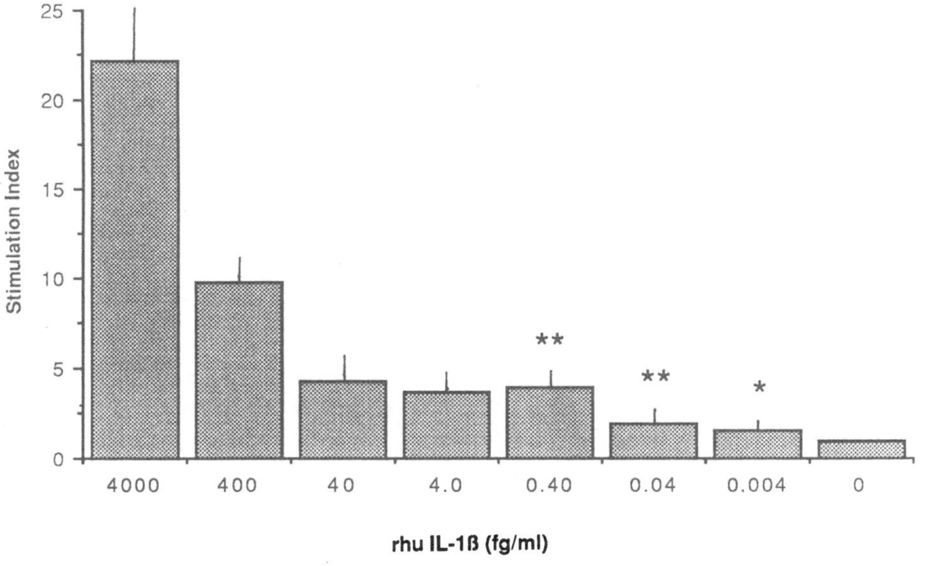

Fig. 1. Proliferative response of D10S cells to rhuIL-1ß in the absence of mitogen. Mean (± SEM) stimulation index of nine experiments. The proliferative response of the control culture without IL-1 was set at 1 and the stimulation index of each concentration of IL-1 was calculated. ** indicates $p<0.001$; * indicates $p<0.01$, Student's unpaired T-test.

represents less than one IL-1 molecule per cell. These results are consistent with those shown in Figure 1.

Specificity of Proliferative Response of D10S Cells

Several recombinant and purified cytokines were tested for their ability to induce proliferation of D10S cells in the presence or absence of mitogen. There were no proliferative responses to several cytokines of human or murine origin used at concentrations 100 to 10,000-fold greater than for IL-1. Proliferation was not observed to endotoxin, human or murine interferon-gamma, human or murine tumor necrosis factor, lymphotoxin, or granulocyte-macrophage colony stimulating factor. There was no suppressive effect of transforming growth factor-beta. Only at high concentrations (100 ng/ml) did human recombinant interleukin-6 induce proliferation.

Of particular interest is the observation that recombinant murine TNF did not induce proliferation in the D10S cells. Recombinant murine TNF does induce a proliferative response in murine thymocytes in the presence of PHA (M. Palladino, personal communication) whereas human TNF has no effect. Purified natural human IL-6 similarly did not induce proliferation, although this material stimulates murine thymocyte proliferation in the presence of PHA.[21] At concentrations of 100 ng/ml, IL-6 induced proliferation comparable to 1 fg/ml of IL-1. When IL-6 was added to D10S cells in the presence of PHA, a similar dose response was observed.

On the other hand, human IL-2 and recombinant murine IL-4 induced proliferation in D10S cells in the absence of mitogen, although on a molar basis, IL-1 was clearly the most active in inducing maximal responses. The D10S subclone does not produce IL-2 or other T-cell growth factors as measured by proliferative responses of murine CTLL cells. Furthermore, we employed specific antibodies to IL-1, IL-2 and IL-4 in order to reduce the proliferative response of D10S cells to each cytokine. In each case, as shown in Figure 2, the specific antibody blocked the proliferative response only to the respective cytokine. These results suggest that each cytokine acts independently as a growth factor for these T-cells.

IL-1 Receptors

Recombinant human IL-1α was labeled with ^{125}I and used for receptor binding studies. The labeled IL-1 binds to the highly sensitive D10S subclone in a specific and saturable manner. Scatchard plot analysis of ^{125}I-IL-1 binding studies at 4C reveals two types of binding sites of high and low affinity. The high affinity binding site has an apparent dissociation constant (Kd) of aboubt 11 pM, with approximately 4800 binding sites per cell. The low affinity binding site has an apparent dissociation constant Kd of about 450 pM and has about 20,000 sites per cell (Figure 3).

By comparison ^{125}IL-1 binds to murine EL4 thymoma cells with a single class of high affinity binding site with an apparent dissociation constant of 55 pM and with about 4000 sites per cell. Both IL-1α and IL-1ß compete for the binding of the radiolabeled IL-1α to its receptor in D10S and EL4 cells. The molecular mass of the receptor molecule on D10S cells is approx. 72 kD by comparison with the approx. 79.5 kD found for the EL4 cells. In addition, D10S cells have a 25 kD binding protein.

When D10S cells are incubated in the presence of IL-1, the IL-1 receptor (IL-1R) undergoes down regulation and the cells display reduced proliferation to IL-1. The effect of interleukin-2 (IL-2) was not always consistent; the IL-1R sites either increased in number or remained unchanged. Interleukin-4 (IL-4) increased the number of IL-1R sites on D10S cells, an effect which was associated with a marked increase of sensitivity of the cells to proliferate to IL-1. Phytohemagglutinin which reduces the proliferation of D10S cells to IL-1 inhibited the binding of IL-1 to these cells at 4C. These results support the concept that the IL-1R on these T-lymphocytes functions as a receptor for the growth-promoting effects of IL-1 and this molecularly distinct IL-1R receptor can be differently modulated by IL-4 or mitogen.

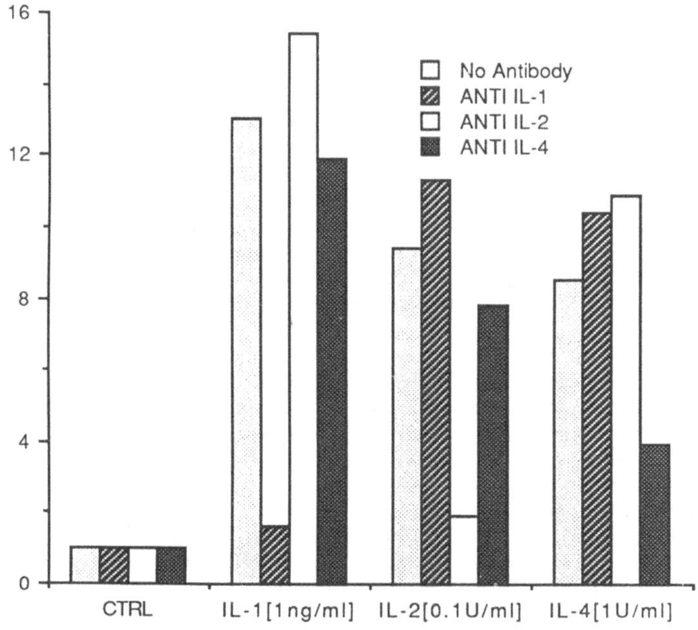

Fig. 2 Effect of different anti-cytokine antibodies on the proliferative responses of D10S cells to either IL-1, IL-2 or IL-4 in the absence of PHA. The concentration of each cytokine used to stimulate the cells is shown under the horizontal axis and the effect of co-incubation with specific antibodie are indicated by the different shadings of the bars. The following cytokine and anti-cytokines were used: rhuIL-1ß and rabbit (0.5% final concentration) anti-IL-1ß; rhuIL-2 and rabbit anti-human IL-2 at 0.5%; rmuIL-4 and monoclonal anti-IL-4 at 30% (v/v).

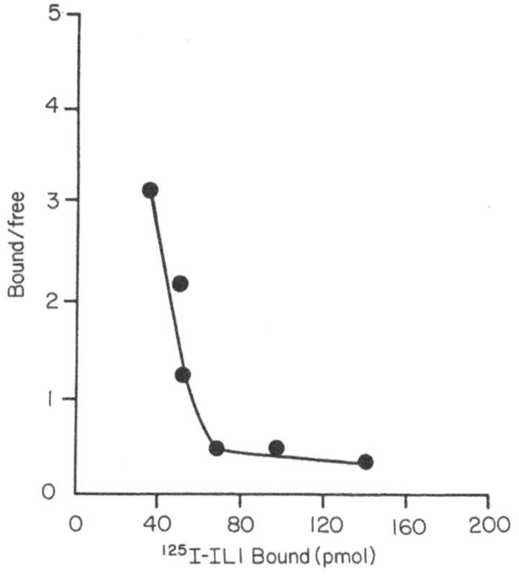

Fig. 3 Scatchard analysis of ^{125}I-IL-1-alpha binding to D10S cells. Cells ($1x10^6$) were incubated overnight at 4°C and the plots represent binding from which non-specific binding (measured in the presence of 50 nM IL-1) has been subtracted.

DISCUSSION

The D10S cells are biologically distinct from the parent D10.G4.1 clone and provide an opportunity to study the direct effect of IL-1 on T-cell proliferation. Previous studies have assigned a "permissive" or "helper" role for IL-1 and T-cell growth. The proliferative response of D10S cells to IL-1 (in the absence of mitogen) places IL-1, together with IL-2 and IL-4, as a direct signal for T-cell growth. Other cytokines do not trigger a proliferative response, even in the presence of mitogen. Of particular importance, we observed no response to several concentrations of TNF (even of murine origin) or lymphotoxin. The proliferative responses to high concentrations (100 ng/ml) of IL-6 suggest that IL-6 may be inducing another lymphokine (IL-1, IL-2 or IL-4) in these cultures.

We show that the direct proliferative response of these cells to IL-1 correlates with IL-1 receptor number and binding affinity. Furthermore, the binding of IL-1 to the D10S cells is significantly higher than that of the parent clone and the response to PHA is reflected in the binding data. The IL-1 receptor on the D10S cells is 1) molecularly distinct from that on EL4 cells, 2) contains two major molecular components, and 3) is down-regulated by mitogen. These characteristics may provide an explanation for the growth-like property of IL-1 for the D10S cells in that these cells have a more complete receptor and hence do not require the signal provided by PMA, mitogen, or calcium ionophores. The EL4 cells have been used extensively to study the IL-1 receptor[5,6,22] and like the parent D10.G4.1 cells, require mitogen or ionophore for optimal response to IL-1.

The proliferative responses of T-cells to IL-1 have demonstrated that IL-1 acts a co-factor, usually with PHA or concanavalin A, whereas in the absence of antigen or mitogen, there is no effect of IL-1 on IL-2 or IL-2 receptor production. Numerous studies of the parent clone of D10.G4.1 cells have yielded similar results, even in recent reports where IL-4 and GM-CSF have been shown to mediate the growth of these cells.[16-18] IL-1 itself is produced by D10.G4.1 cells[23] and that cell-associated IL-1 may participate in antigen recognition of these cells. In a recent study, the function of IL-1 to act as a co-factor for a proliferative signal, which can be replaced by substances that activate protein kinases, was mimicked by 1,25-dihydroxy vitamin D-3.[24]

A consistent pattern of the proliferative response of the D10S clone is that the presence of PHA suppresses the response. This was even observed when high concentrations of recombinant human IL-6 were used. This biological property sets these cells apart from the parent clone. As shown in the accompanying paper, receptor binding for IL-1 on the D10S cells is reduced by exposure to low (1 ug/ml) concentrations of PHA. This relationship of receptor number or binding to the measured proliferative response was also observed with prior incubation of the D10S cells with either IL-1 or IL-4. Thus IL-1 appears to act as a direct growth factor for these cells in relationship to the numbers of IL-1 receptors. This latter concept is supported by the experiments in which the cells were exposed to IL-1 for different periods of time. If IL-1 was acting as an inducer of another growth factor, then its effect on these cells would take place early during stimulation. However, as shown using either the introduction of specific anti-IL-1 or the addition of IL-1 at different time points, proliferation was direct consequence of the presence of IL-1.

Although we cannot exclude the induction of another factor or receptor for such a factor as a mechanism for IL-1 on these cells, the data suggest that IL-1 provides a direct proliferative signal for these cells. Since D10.G4.1 cells can produce IL-1,[23] IL-1 may be acting as a growth factor during the time of antigen presentation, but after several days, the cells become IL-1 dependent and exhibit a dramatic proliferative response to subfemtomolar concentrations of the cytokine.

A role for IL-4 (B-cell stimulating factor-1) as a growth factor for D10.G4.1 cells has received recent attention.[16,17] Upon stimulation with antigen, D10.G4.1 cells produce another B-cell growth factor which increases the proliferation of large B-cells and synergizes with human B-cell growth factor for optimal secretion of IgM.[25] In a cloned murine Th2 cell line, IL-1 plus ionomycin induced IL-4 production and proliferation in these cells was shown to be dependent on the elaboration of IL-4.[26] However, using phorbol esters as a co-stimulant, these cells proliferated to IL-1 independent of IL-4 elaboration. In general, IL-4 as a direct autocrine growth factor appears to be well-established for some T-cell lines. However, we were unable to show that monoclonal anti-IL-4 reduced the proliferative response of the D10S cells to IL-1. Furthermore, the negative effect of mitogens on the proliferation of these cells to IL-1 is in direct contrast to all the published reports for observing the optimal conditions for both proliferation as well as elaboration of IL-4 in D10.G4.1 and Th2 type cells.

Recently, several subclones of the D10.G4.1 cell line have been made using the Kirsten murine sarcoma virus,[27], and the ras-expressing transfectants proliferate to IL-1 is the absence of mitogen, similar to the D10S cells. Also similar to the D10S cells, the ability of these transfectants to proliferate to IL-1 is independent of IL-4. Like the parent clone, these virally infected cells proliferate to IL-2 but their response to IL-1 is not through production of IL-2. However, the ras expressing D10.G4.1 cells demonstrate the typical augmentation of proliferation when IL-1 and mitogen are used together. This finding distinguishes our clone from the ras expressing cells. Nevertheless, purposeful infection with the murine sarcoma virus results in expression of viral oncogenes which apparently allows these cells independence of IL-2 and IL-4, yet at the same time, sensitive to the sole proliferative effect of IL-1. We can only speculate at the present time that our subclone may have been accidentally infected with a retrovirus and is similar to those cells described by Lichtman. Furthermore, it is possible that the "growth factor" property of IL-1 for our clone represents the ability of IL-1 to trigger an oncogene product that functions as a novel receptor of IL-1.

Another variant of the D10.G4.1 cell line also seems similar to the D10S cells. Designated MD10 cells,[28] these cells bear the parent clonotypic antigen receptor (3D3) but proliferate to low doses of IL-1 (fM). Like the D10S cells, MD10 cells proliferation to IL-1 is maximal at 72 hours and is not inhibited by anti-IL-4. Although like D10S cells, the MD10 cells could possibly release an intermediate growth factor, this was not detected using either CTLL or HT-2 cells. The authors concluded that MD10 cells respond to IL-1 like a growth factor and we believe that the D10S cells similarly proliferate to IL-1 directly. We have recently observed proliferation of D10S cells which have been repeatedly cultured without accessory cells or antigen. It is possible that these cells are providing their own growth factor or IL-1 itself[23] which then acts as growth factor.

ACKNOWLEDGMENTS

We thank Dr. W.E. Paul for the anti-IL-4 antibody and Dr. C.A. Janeway, Jr., for the original D10.G4.1 clone. Also, we thank Dr. Takashi Ikejima for the CTLL cells and Dr. Lanny J. Rosenwasser a parent clone of the D10.G4.1.

REFERENCES

1. C.A. Dinarello, The biology of interleukin-1, FASEB J 2:108 (1988).
2. C.A. Dinarello, T. Ikejima, S.J.C. Warner, S.F. Orencole, G. Lonnemann, J.G. Cannon, and P. Libby, Interleukin-1 induces interleukin-1. I. Induction of circulating interleukin-1 in rabbits in vivo and in human mononuclear cells in vitro, J immunol 139:1902 (1987).
3. B. Beutler and A. Cerami, Cachectin and tumor necrosis factor as two sides of the same biolocial coin, Nature 320:584 (1986).
4. T.A. Bird, A.J.H. Gearing, and J. Saklatvala, Murine interleukin-1 receptor: difference in binding properties between fibroblastic and thymoma cells and evidence for a two-chain receptor model, FEBS Lett 225:21 (1987).

5. P.O. Kilian, K.L. Kaffka, A.S. Stern, D. Woehle, W.R. Benjamin, T.M. DeChiara, U. Gubler, J.J. Farrar, S.B. Mizel, and P.T. Lomedico, Interleukin-1-alpha and interleukin-1-beta bind to the same receptor on T cells, J Immunol 136:4509 (1986).
6. J.W. Lowenthal and H.R. MacDonald, Binding and internalization of interleukin-1 by T cells. Direct evidence for high and low affinity classes of interleukin-1 receptor, J Exp Med 164:1060 (1986).
7. K. Matsushima, J. Yodoi, Y. Tagaya and J.J. Oppenheim, Down-regulation of interleukin-1 (IL-1) receptor expression by IL-1 and fate of internalized ^{125}I-labeled IL-1-beta in a human large granular lymphocyte cell line, J Immunol 137:3183 (1986).
8. F. Shirakawa, Y. Tanaka, T. Ota, H. Suzuki, S. Eto, and U. Yamashita, Expression of interleukin-1 receptors on human peripheral T cells, J Immunol 138:4243 (1987).
9. S.B. Mizel, Interleukin-1 and T cell activation, Immunol Rev 63:51 (1982).
10. S.K. Durum, J.A. Schmidt, and J.J. Oppenheim, Interleukin-1: an immunological perspective. Ann Rev Immunol 3:263 (1985).
11. T. Krakauer, D. Mizel, and J.J. Oppenheim, Independent and synergistic thymocyte proliferative activities of PMA and IL-1, J. Immunol. 129:939 (1982).
12. P.L. Simon, Calcium mediates one of the signals required for interleukin-1 and 2 production by murine cell lines, Cell Immunol 87:720 (1984).
13. K.A. Smith, L.B. Lachman, J.J. Oppenheim, and M.F. Favata, The functional relationship of the interleukins, J Exp Med 151:1551 (1980).
14. J.M. Williams, D. DeLoria, J.A. Hansen, C.A. Dinarello, R. Loertxcher, H.M. Shapiro, and T.B. Strom, The events of primary T cell activation can be staged by use of sepharose-bound anti-T3 (64.1) monoclonal antibody and purified interleukin-1, J. Immunol. 135:2249 (1985).
15. J. Kaye, S. Gillis, S.B. Mizel, E.M. Shevach, T.R. Malek, C.A. Dinarello, L.B. Lachman, and C.A. Janeway, Jr., Growth of a cloned helper T-cell line induced by a monoclonal antibody specific for the antigen receptor: interleukin-1 is required for the expression of receptors for interleukin-2. J. Immunol. 133:1339 (1984).
16. A.H. Lichtman, E.A. Kurt-Jones, and A.K. Abbas, B cell stimulatory factor 1 and not interleukin-2 is the autocrine growth factor for some helper T lymphocytes, Proc. Natl. Acad. Sci. USA 84:824 (1987).
17. T. Kupper, M. Horowitz, F. Lee, R. Robb and P.M. Flood, Autocrine growth of T cells independent of interleukin-2: identification of interleukin-4 (IL-4, BSF-1) as an autocrine growth factor for a cloned antigen-specific helper T cell. J. Immunol. 138: 4280.
18. T. Kupper, P. Flood, D. Coleman, and M. Horowitz, Growth of an interleukin 2/interleukin 4-dependent T cell line induced by granulocyte-macrophage colony-stimulating factor (GM-CSF), J. Immunol. 138:4288 (1987).
19. G. Lonnemann, S. Endres, J.W.M. van der Meer, J.G. Cannon, and C.A. Dinarello, A radioimmunoassay for production from human mononuclear cells. Lymphokine Res. (in press).
20. J. Ohara and W.E. Paul, Production of a monoclonal antibody to and molecular characterization of B-cell stimulating factor-1, Nature 315:333 (1985).
21. A. Billiau, BSF-2 is not just a differentiation factor, Nature 324:415 (1986).
22. J.W. Lowenthal, J.-C. Cerottini, and H.R. MacDonald, Interleukin-1 dependent induction of both interleukin-2 secretion and interleukin-2 receptor expression by thymoma cells, J Immunol 137:1226 (1986).
23. B. Tartakovsky, E.J. Kovacs, L. Takacs, and S.K. Durum, T cell clone producing an IL-1-like activity after stimulation by antigen-presenting B cells. J. Immunol. 137:160 (1986).
24. D.L. Lacey, J. Axelrod, J.C. Chappel, A.J. Kahn, and S.L. Teitelbaum, Vitamin D affects proliferation of a murine T helper cell clone, J. Immunol. 138:1680 (1987).
25. D.L. Ennist, K.L. Elkins, S.C. Cheng, and M. Howard, Activity of a partially purified human BCGF on murine assays for B cell stimulatory factors. II. Synergy between two distinct BCGF II-like factors in promoting B cell differentiation, J. Immunol. 139:1525 (1987).

26. S. Ho, R.T. Abraham, A. Nilson, B.S. Handwerger, and D.J. McKean, Interleukin-1-mediated activation of interleukin-4 producing T lymphocytes. Proliferation by IL-4-dependent and IL-4-independent mechanisms. J. Immunol. 139:1532 (1987).
27. A.H. Lichtman, M.E. Williams, J. Ohara, W.E. Paul, D.V. Faller, and A.K. Abbas, Retrovirus infection alters growth factor responses of T lymphocytes, J. Immunol. 138:3276 (1987).
28. D.L. Lacey, J.C. Chappel, S.L. Teitelbaum, Interleukin-1 stimulates proliferation of a nontransformed T lymphocyte line in the absence of co-mitogen, J. Immunol. 139:2649 (1987).

STRUCTURE AND REGULATION OF THE HUMAN IL-2 RECEPTOR

Warner C. Greene, Ernst Böhnlein, Miriam Siekevitz*, Dean W. Ballard, B. Robert Franza+and John W. Lowenthal

Howard Hughes Medical Institute, Box 3037 Duke University Medical Center, Durham, North Carolina
*Mt. Sinai Medical Center, One Gustave Levy Place, New York, New York
+Cold Spring Harbor Laboratory, P.O. Box 534, Cold Spring Harbor, New York

INTRODUCTION

The growth of human T lymphocytes can be divided into two discrete stages resembling competence and progression. In the first stage, the binding of antigen or mitogen to specific T cell receptors triggers the transduction of intracellular signals leading to cellular activation[1, 2]. In turn, these activation signals induce the de novo expression of genes mediating T cell growth including interleukin-2 (IL-2) and interleukin-2 receptors (IL-2R)[3-5]. The subsequent binding of IL-2 to its high affinity receptor promotes proliferation and clonal expansion of the cells originally stimulated by antigen.

IL-2 RECEPTOR STRUCTURE

Three different forms of the human IL-2R have now been identified including high, intermediate, and low affinity binding sites. The high affinity IL-2R appear to correspond to a membrane receptor complex composed of at least two IL-2 binding subunits including the well-characterized 55 kD Tac antigen (p55,IL-2Rα)[6, 7] and a recently recognized 70-75 kD protein (p70, IL-2Rß)[8-12]. These high affinity receptors interact with IL-2 with an apparent K_d of 2-20 pM and appear to be the primary receptor form responsible for mediating the growth-promoting response to IL-2. The intermediate affinity IL-2 receptors correspond to the IL-2Rß protein alone. This receptor binds ligand with an apparent K_d of 0.5-1.0. nM[10-12] and in the presence of high concentrations of IL-2 appears capable of transducing intracellular signals. The low affinity receptors are formed by the IL-2Rα protein expressed in the absence of IL-2Rß subunit[9, 12, 13]. These receptors bind IL-2 with a K_d of 10-20nM[13]. Recent studies suggest that the IL-2Rα and IL-2Rß proteins interact with different epitopes on the IL-2 molecule[11] thus providing a rational explanation for high affinity binding by the α -ß heterodimeric complex of proteins.

Additional studies have revealed that the kinetics of IL-2 association and dissociation from these individual receptor subunits are strikingly different[14, 15]. Specifically, IL-2 rapidly associates with the IL-2Rα protein with a $t_{1/2}$ of approximately 5 seconds. However, this receptor binds ligand with low affinity due to the rapid dissociation of ligand with a $t_{1/2}$ of 5-10 seconds[14, 15]. In sharp contrast, IL-2 associates with the IL-2Rß protein with remarkably slower kinetics displaying a $t_{1/2}$ of 40-50 minutes[14, 15]. This slow rate of association suggests that this process may not be solely limited by ligand diffusion but rather may involve conformational changes in receptor structure. Once IL-2 has bound to the IL-2Rß protein, it dissociates very slowly with a measured $t_{1/2}$ of 4-5 hours[14, 15] thus explaining the intermediate affinity of these binding sites. Interestingly, the high affinity receptor displays a composite of these association and dissociation kinetics[14, 15]. The on rate for IL-2 binding to the high affinity receptor occurs with a $t_{1/2}$ of approximately 30 seconds resembling the rapid association rate characteristic of the IL-2Rα chain[14,15]. In contrast, the off rate is quite slow occurring with a $t_{1/2}$ of about 4 hours which is very similar to slow dissociation of ligand from the IL-2Rß chain[14, 15]. These findings underscore the important contributions of each individual subunit to the assembly of a receptor complex uniquely able to rapidly bind and retain its ligand.

Recent studies also have shown that the IL-2Rß protein alone is capable of mediating rapid endocytosis of ligand in a manner essentially identical to the high affinity receptor[16]. In contrast, the IL-2Rα protein is incapable of internalizing IL-2. As the intracytoplasmic domains of proteins largely regulate endocytosis, these findings suggest that the cytoplasmic region of IL-2Rß may be larger than the 13 residues present in the IL-2Rα chain[17].

Constitutive surface expression of the IL-2Rß protein in the absence of IL-2Rα subunit has recently been detected in resting T cells[12, 18] and natural killer cells[12, 19-21]. In the presence of large quantities of IL-2, the interaction of ligand with these intermediate affinity IL-2Rß receptors appears to transduce signals leading to the activation of resting T cells[18] and increased cytolytic activity in the natural killer cells[21]. Interestingly, with both cell types, IL-2 binding to the IL-2Rß protein activates IL-2Rα gene expression ultimately leading to the assembly of high affinity IL-2 receptors[18, 21] which in some cases appear to mediate the proliferative response. At present, the structure of the IL-2Rß protein remains unknown. Importantly, it is unknown whether the receptor subunit contains tyrosine kinase activity characteristic of many other growth factor receptors. Notwithstanding, it seems likely that this subunit plays a central role in signal transduction mediated by the high affinity receptor. Further study is required to determine if high affinity binding involves a stable association of the IL-2Rα and IL-2Rß chains as convincing evidence for a ternary complex of IL-2 and the receptor subunits has not yet been obtained. The molecular cloning of IL-2Rß cDNAs may provide important clues to the long elusive mechanism of high affinity receptor signal transduction.

Recently, our investigations have focused on the regulation of IL-2Rα gene expression as its rapid induction following mitogen stimulation plays an important role in the assembly of high affinity IL-2R. The 5' flanking region of the IL-2Rα gene has been cloned, sequenced and analyzed both for the location of cis-acting sequences required for mitogen activation[22-25] and for the potential interaction of trans-acting nuclear proteins with these regulatory sequences[25, 26]. To define sequences required for mitogen activation, a processively deleted series of the IL-2Rα promoter mutants were prepared with Bal 31 and positioned in correct orientation immediately upstream of the chloramphenicol acetyltransferase (CAT) reporter gene. These expression plasmids were thentransfected into various lymphoid cell lines, and the cultures activated with different inducing agents[25]. In Jurkat T cells, we observed that -317 pTacCAT plasmids (numbering relative to the major distal cap site at +1) were fully activated by PHA or PMA while -271 pTacCAT plasmids were virtually inactive. In sharp contrast, -271 pTacCAT plasmids were readily induced by PMA, IL-1, or forskolin in the immature YT-1 leukemic T cell line while -179 pTacCAT constructs were inactive. In Jurkat T cells, the -271 pTacCAT plasmid was readily induced by the transactivator (tax-1) gene product of HTLV-1 but not by PHA or PMA[23, 25]. Thus, the requisite promoter sequences appear to differ depending upon the nature of the inducing signal and perhaps the state of cellular maturation.

Two imperfect direct repeats (IDRs) were detected within the IL-2Rα promoter sequence immediately flanking base -271. Since such repetitive elements have been implicated in the binding of transcriptional factors in other systems, we investigated whether this region of the IL-2Rα promoter was involved in DNA-protein interactions[25, 26]. Three different double stranded oligonucleotides were synthesized and used in gel retardation assays. The IL-2R I oligonucleotide contained sequences spanning the upstream IDR region, the IL-2R II oligonucleotide contained sequences associated with the downstream IDR region, while the IL-2R III oligonucleotide contained sequences spanning both of these IDRs. Using the IL-2R III probe, we found that nuclear proteins from PHA or PMA stimulated, but not unstimulated, Jurkat T cells formed two retarded DNA-protein complexes[25]. The formation of these DNA-protein complexes was specific as unlabeled IL-2R III blocked their appearance while a size-matched oligonucleotide from the ampicillin resistance gene of pBR322 did not. These two retarded complexes were also detectable using nuclear extracts from Jurkat cells expressing the tax-1 protein of HTLV-1, tax-1 producing leukemic cells, and YT cells stimulated with PMA, or PMA and forskolin[25].

Competition studies with different oligonucleotides were next performed to localize the binding site(s) involved in complex formation[25]. The IL-2R II oligonucleotide containing sequences corresponding to the downstream IDR completely blocked the formation of both complexes with the IL-2R III oligonucleotide. In contrast, the IL-2R I oligonucleotide containing sequences from the upstream IDR region was not inhibitory. In direct binding assays, the IL-2R II probe formed one DNA-protein complex with induced Jurkat nuclear extracts, but two complexes with induced YT nuclear extracts. This finding paralleled the functional assays where sequences upstream of -271 were required for mitogen activation in Jurkat cells but not in YT-1 cells.

To identify the precise protein binding site within the IL-2R II probe, a series of mutated versions of IL-2R II were prepared and tested for competitive effects and direct binding activity[26]. This approach permitted localization of the binding site to a 12 bp region between nucleotides -265 and -256. Ortho-phenanthroline copper footprinting confirmed protein binding in this region. Comparison of the sequence of this putative IL-2Rα promoter region with other known DNA binding sites revealed a striking similarity to the enhancer element of the type I human immunodeficiency virus (HIV-1) and the enhancer of the kappa light chain immunoglobulin enhancer[27]. This sequence homology proved functionally significant as unlabelled HIV-1 enhancer oligonucleotides completely blocked the binding of proteins to the IL-2Rα promoter[26]. Similarly, the IL-2Rα promoter oligonucleotides blocked the formation of at least two inducible DNA protein complexes with the HIV-1 enhancer. Direct evidence for the binding of the same inducible nuclear protein to both the IL-2Rα promoter and HIV-1 enhancer was obtained using a DNA affinity precipitation assay[26, 28]. Nuclear proteins from induced or uninduced Jurkat cells were radiolabeled with ^{35}S-methionine and then incubated either with biotinylated wild-type or mutant oligonucleotide probes from the IL-2Rα promoter and the HIV-I enhancer[26]. DNA-protein complexes were precipitated with avidin-agarose and the eluted proteins analyzed on high resolution 2-dimensional polyacrylamide gels. Both the wild-type HIV-1 enhancer and IL-2Rα promoter wild-type oligonucleotides specifically complexed with an 86kD inducible protein termed HIVEN86A[26, 28]. In contrast, an IL-2Rα promoter oligonucleotide mutated within the 12 bp binding site failed to interact with this inducible transcriptional factor. These findings confirmed that both the HIV-1 enhancer and IL-2Rα promoter shared the binding of at least one common inducible nuclear protein.

These results provided a potential explanation for the observation that the HIV-1 LTR is activated by the same mitogens (ionomycin, PHA, PMA, and tax-1)[27, 29-31] that activate the IL-2Rα promoter[22-25, 32]. Deletion analysis of the HIV-1 LTR has revealed that the enhancer element played an important role[29-31] although additional upstream regulatory elements contributed in both a positive and negative manner to the overall level of the response[29]. The HIV-1 enhancer alone was found to be sufficient to impart mitogen inducibility to the mitogen insensitive thymidine kinase (TK) promoter[29, 31]. Nabel and Baltimore[27] had previously reported that a nuclear factor indistinguishable from NF-κB interacted with the HIV-1 enhancer. At present, the relationship of HIVEN86A to NF-κB remains unclear. It is possible that HIVEN86A[28] and NF-κB correspond to the same protein or perhaps that HIVEN86A is a member of an NF-κB family of proteins. Alternatively, these factors may represent different proteins that share a common binding site specificity. Of interest, NF-κB activity has been detected in non-lymphoid HeLa cells following activation with PMA[27]. In view of this finding, we tested whether the IL-2Rα promoter and HIV-1 enhancer could be activated by PMA in HeLa cells[26]. Transfection studies revealed that the IL-2Rα promoter was inactive in these cells either in the presence or absence of PMA. The TK promoter modified with the HIV-1 enhancer also was not inducible by PMA in HeLa cells, however, considerable constitutive activity compared to the unmodified TK promoter alone was evident. In contrast to the lack of mitogen induction in HeLa cells, both the IL-2Rα promoter and HIV-1 enhancer were markedly activated by PMA in Jurkat or YT-1 T cells. These findings suggested the possible involvement of a lymphoid specific factor. Consistent with this notion, gel retardation assays with IL-2R III or the HIV-1 enhancer and nuclear extracts from PMA induced HeLa cells revealed a single complex in contrast to two specific complexes with extracts from PMA induced Jurkat T cells. Of interest, the HIVEN86A protein has not been detected in induced HeLa cells (B.R. Franza: unpublished data). Thus, it is possible that this protein might represent a restricting element accounting for the tissue specific nature of IL-2Rα gene expression. However, additional biochemical analyses are required to resolve the relationship of the HIVEN86A protein to the NF-κB activities present in induced T cells and HeLa cells.

While the activation of IL-2Rα gene expression is involved in the promotion of T cell growth and the activation of HIV-1 gene replication is commonly associated with T cell death, these diverse responses appear to be initially regulated by the same inducible 86kD nuclear transcription factor. The activation of the HIV-I LTR by mitogens may play an important role in controlling whether the infection occurs in a latent or lytic manner. The design of therapeutic agents capable of interfering with enhancer dependent HIV-1 LTR stimulation might inhibit the activation of latent virus and the cell death associated with retroviral replication. However, these drugs must also be carefully evaluated for their potential effects on the activation of a variety of genes involved in normal T cell growth including the IL-2Rα gene.

REFERENCES

1. A. Weiss, J. Imboden, D. Schoback, and J. Stobo. 1984. Role of T3 surface molecules in the activation of human T cells: T3 dependent activation results in a rise in cytoplasmic free calcium. Proc. Natl. Acad. Sci. USA 81:4169-4173.
2. A. Weiss and J.B. Imboden. 1987. Cell surface molecules and early events involved in human T lymphocyte activation. Adv. Immunol. 41:1-38.
3. T. Taniguchi, H. Matsui, T. Fujita, M. Hatakeyama, N. Kashima, A. Fuse, J. Hamuro, C. Nishi-Takaoka and G. Yamada. 1986. Molecular analysis of the interleukin-2 and its cellular receptor. Prog. Hematol. 14:283-301.
4. W.C. Greene, W.J. Leonard, and J.M. Depper. 1986. Growth of human T lymphocytes: an analysis of interleukin-2 and its cellular receptor. Prog. Hematol. 14:283-301.
5. K.A. Smith. 1984. Interleukin 2. Ann. Rev. Immunol. 2:319-333.
6. W.J. Leonard, J.M. Depper, R.J. Robb, T.A. Waldmann, and W.C. Greene. 1982. A monoclonal antibody that appears to recognize the receptor for human T-cell growth factor. Nature 300:267-269.
7. R.J. Robb and W.C. Greene. 1983. Direct demonstration of the identity of T cell growth factor binding protein and the Tac antigen. J. Exp. Med. 158: 1332-1337.
8. M. Sharon, R.D. Klausner, B.R. Cullen, R. Chizzonite and W.J. Leonard. 1986. Novel interleukin-2 receptor subunit detected by cross-linking under high-affinity conditions. Science 234:859-863.
9. M. Tsudo, R.W. Kozak, C.K. Goldman, and T.A. Waldmann. 1986. Demonstration of a non-Tac peptide that binds interleukin 2: a potential participant in a multichain interleukin 2 receptor complex. Proc. Natl. Acad. Sci. 83:9694-9698.
10. K. Teshigawara, H.M. Wang, K. Kato and K.A. Smith. 1987. Interleukin 2 high-affinity receptor expression requires two distinct binding proteins. J. Exp. Med. 165:223-238.

11. R.J. Robb, C.M. Rusk, J. Yodoi and W.C. Greene. 1987. Interleukin 2 binding molecule distinct from the Tac protein: analysis of its role in formation of high-affinity receptors. Proc. Natl. Acad. Sci. 84:2002-2006.
12. M. Dukovich, Y. Wano, L. Thuy, P. Katz, B.R. Cullen, J.H. Kehrl and W.C. Greene. 1987. A second human interleukin-2 binding protein that may be a component of high-affinity interleukin-2 receptors. Nature 327:518-522.
13. M. Fujii, K. Sugamura, K. Sano, M. Nakai, K. Sugita and Y. Hinuma. 1986. High-affinity receptor mediated internalization and degradation of interleukin 2 in human T cells. J. Exp. Med. 163:550-555.
14. J.W. Lowenthal, and W.C. Greene. 1987. Contrasting interleukin 2 binding properties of the α (p55) and ß (p70) protein subunits of the human high affinity interleukin 2 receptor. J. Exp. Med. 166:1156-1161.
15. H.-M. Wang, and K.A. Smith. 1987. The interleukin 2 receptor: functional consequences of its bimolecular structure. J. Exp. Med. 166:1055-1069.
16. R.J. Robb, and W.C. Greene. 1987. Internalization of interleukin 2 is mediated by the ß chain of the high affinity interleukin 2 receptor. J. Exp. Med. 165:1202-1212.
17. W.J. Leonard, J.M. Depper, G.R. Crabtree, S. Rudikoff, J. Pumphrey, R. Robb, M. Kronke, P.B. Svetlik, N.J. Peffer, T.A. Waldmann and W.C. Greene. 1984. Molecular cloning and expression of cDNAs for the human interleukin-2 receptor. Nature 311:626-631.
18. Le thi Bich-Thuy, M. Dukovich, N.J. Peffer, A.S. Fauci, J.H. Kehrl and W.C. Greene. 1987. Direct activation of human T cells by IL-2: the role of an IL-2 receptor distinct from the Tac protein. J. Immunol. 139(5):1550-1556.
19. M. Tsudo, C.K. Goldman, K.F. Bongiovanni, W.C. Chan, E.F. Winton, M. Yagita, E.A. Grimm and T.A. Waldmann. 1987. The p75 peptide is the receptor for interleukin 2 expressed on large granular lymphocytes and is responsible for the interleukin 2 activation of these cells. Proc. Natl. Acad. Sci. USA. 84:5394-8.
20. J.P. Siegel, M. Sharon, P.L. Smith and W.J. Leonard. 1987. The IL-2 receptor beta chain (p70): role in mediating signals for LAK, NK, and proliferative activities. Science 238:75-78.
21. J.H. Kehrl, M. Dukovich, G. Whalen, P. Katz, A.S. Fauci and W.C. Greene. 1988. Novel interleukin-2 (IL-2) receptor appears to mediate IL-2 induced activation of natural killer cells. J. Clinical. Invest. 81:200-205.
22. M. Maruyama, H. Shibuya, H. Harada, M. Hatakeyama, M. Seiki, T. Fujita, J. Inoue, M. Yoshida and T. Taniguchi. 1987. Evidence for aberrant activation of the interleukin-2 autocrine loop by HTLV-I-encoded $p40^x$ and T3/Ti complex triggering. Cell 48:343-350.
23. S.L. Cross, M.B. Feinberg, J.B. Wolf, N.J. Holbrook. F. Wong-Staal and W.J. Leonard. 1987. Regulation of the human interleukin-2 receptor chain promoter: activation of a nonfunctional promoter by the transactivator gene of HTLV I. Cell 49:47-56.
24. N. Suzuki, N. Matsunami, H. Kanamori, N. Ishida, A. Shimizu, Y. Yaoita, T. Nikaido and T. Honjo. 1987. The human IL-2 receptor gene contains a positive regulatory element that functions in cultured cells and cell-free extracts. J. Biol. Chem. 262:5079-5086
25. J.W. Lowenthal, E. Böhnlein, D.W. Ballard and W.C. Greene. 1988. Regulation of IL-2 receptor α subunit (Tac) gene expression: binding of inducible nuclear proteins to discrete promoter sequences correlates with transcriptional activation. Proc. Natl. Acad. Sci. USA 85: 4468-4472.
26. E. Böhnlein, E., J.W. Lowenthal, M. Siekevitz, D.W. Ballard, B.R. Franza and W.C. Greene. 1988. The same inducible transcription factor regulates mitogen induced activation of the interleukin-2 receptor gene and type 1 human immunodeficiency virus. Cell 53: 827-836.
27. G. Nabel and D. Baltimore. 1987. An inducible transcription factor activates expression of human immunodeficiency virus in T cells. Nature 326:711-783.
28. R.B. Franza, S.F. Josephs, M.Z. Gilman, W. Ryan and B. Clarkson. 1987. Characterization of cellular proteins recognizing the HIV enhancer using a microscale DNA-affinity precipitation assay. Nature 330:391-395.

29. M. Siekevitz, M., S.F. Josephs, M. Dukovich, N. Peffer, F. Wong-Staal and W.C. Greene. 1987b. Activation of the HIV-1 LTR by T-cell mitogens and the tax-I protein of HTLV-I. Science 238:1575-1578.
30. J.D. Kaufman, G. Valandra, G. Rodriguez, G. Bushar, C. Giri and M.D. Norcross. 1987. Phorbol ester enhances human immunodeficiency virus-promoted gene expression and acts on a repeated 10-base-pair functional enhancer element. Molec. Cell Biol. 7:3759-3766.
31. S.E. Tong-Starksen, P.A. Luciw and B.M. Peterlin. Human immunodeficiency virus long terminal repeat responds to T-cell activation signals. Proc. Natl. Acad. Sci. 84:6845-6849.
32. M. Siekevitz, M.B. Feinberg, N. Holbrook, J. Yodoi, F. Wong-Staal and W.C. Greene. 1987a. Activation of interleukin-2 and interleukin-2 receptor (Tac) promoter expression by the trans-activator (tax) gene product of human T-cell leukemia virus, type I. Proc. Natl. Acad. Sci. 84:5389-5393.

STRUCTURE-FUNCTION RELATIONSHIPS FOR HIGH AND LOW-AFFINITY INTERLEUKIN 2 RECEPTORS

Richard J. Robb

Medical Products Department
E. I. du Pont de Nemours & Co.
Glenolden, PA 19036

INTRODUCTION

The original study of interleukin 2 (IL-2) binding to activated lymphocytes by Robb and colleagues[1] described a high-affinity receptor-ligand association which fit nicely with the very low levels of IL-2 which promoted cellular proliferation. Later studies, however, demonstrated that the IL-2 receptor actually existed in a number of forms with drastically different affinities for ligand[2]. Our subsequent research has focused on explaining these differences in molecular terms and relating them to the function of this versatile growth and differentiation factor. Insight into structure-function relationships for the IL-2-receptor system should prove particularly valuable to the design of drugs which can be used to manipulate IL-2-dependent immunological responses.

MULTIPLE FORMS OF THE IL-2 RECEPTOR

Based on our own work and that of other investigators, it appears that at least two distinct cell-surface proteins are capable of specifically binding IL-2[3-6]. When they are present alone, these proteins bind IL-2 with a low or intermediate affinity. When they are present together on the same cell, however, a high-affinity receptor binding site is formed. Thus, at least three forms of IL-2 receptors exist which differ in their subunit composition and ligand affinity.

Type I Receptors - The Tac Receptor Chain

Activation of human lymphocytes by antigens, lectins and certain viruses results in the surface expression of a 55,000 m.w. glycoprotein termed Tac[7]. The Tac protein is expressed in both high (K_d ~5 to 20 pM) and low-affinity (K_d ~ 10 to 20 nM) configurations. A variety of experimental data indicates that this difference is due to the presence in high-affinity binding sites of a second receptor subunit[8-11]. Thus, by itself, Tac binds IL-2 with a low affinity. Such low-affinity receptors fail to internalize ligand and may be incapable of mediating any IL-2-dependent cellular response[12]. As an integral component of the molecular complex which constitutes high-affinity receptors, however, the Tac protein plays a crucial role in increasing the sensitivity of activated lymphocytes to IL-2.

The interaction of the Tac protein and IL-2 provides an opportunity for modulating cellular responses to IL-2 which are mediated by high-affinity receptors. Since localization of the binding sites on the two molecules would be useful in the design of IL-2 agonists and antagonists, we have conducted a series of experiments aimed at identifying the contact sites of this interaction. Crosslinking studies demonstrated that low-affinity Tac receptors combined with IL-2 in a one-to-one stoichiometry to form a 70,000 m.w. complex. Proteolytic fragmentation of this complex demonstrated that IL-2 was covalently linked to a lysine amino group within the N-terminal 83 positions of the Tac molecule[13]. Thus, segments of the receptor protein encoded by exons 2 (residues 1-64) and 3 (residues 65-101) of the Tac gene appeared to be involved in contact with the ligand. Amino acids present in the segment encoded by exon 4 (residues 102 to 173) also appeared essential, however, since deletion of this exon from a cDNA clone of the Tac molecule resulted in the synthesis of an inactive protein product[14].

The requirement for exon 4-encoded residues for an active Tac protein may be explained in part by the contribution of intramolecular disulfide bonding. A preliminary map of the disulfide bonds of the Tac protein based on analysis of cystine-linked peptide fragments indicated that Cys 3 (exon 2) and Cys 147 (exon 4) were joined[15]. Site-specific mutagenesis of either of these two Cys led to the synthesis of an inactive protein which was not properly exported from the endoplasmic reticulum. Deletion of exon 4 from the cDNA clone would have similarly prevented the formation of this bond, resulting in an improperly-folded protein. In addition to the linkage of Cys 3 and 147, disulfide bonds appeared to connect Cys 28,30 with Cys 59,61, Cys 131 with Cys 163 and Cys 46 with Cys 104. Substitution of Ala for Cys at any of these positions caused the protein to fold improperly. The location and contribution of these disulfide bonds emphasizes the interdependence of the protein segments encoded by exons 2 and 4 of the Tac gene.

The interdependence of the exon 2 and exon 4-encoded protein regions raises doubts as to whether a short contiguous segment of Tac protein residues can bind IL-2 with a significant affinity. In fact, we found that the shortest form of the Tac molecule capable of normal ligand interaction consisted of the N-terminal 163 amino acids[15]. Truncated versions of the protein terminating at various locations in the exon 3 segment and at the beginning of the exon 4 region were inactive. Nevertheless, site-specific mutagenesis of the Tac protein indicated that parts of the IL-2 binding site could be mapped to two, and perhaps as many as four, discrete segments within the first 163 amino acid positions. Two of these segments coincided with the epitopes of anti-Tac monoclonal antibodies which blocked IL-2 binding, making them likely candidates for actual ligand-receptor contact sites. This information provides a rational basis for beginning to design IL-2 analogues and should be particularly useful in interpreting crystallographic analyses of the Tac protein.

Type II Receptors - The Beta Receptor Chain

Several reports describing the effect of IL-2 on natural killer (NK) cells and a particular B cell line suggested the existence of an IL-2 receptor which did not contain the Tac protein[16,17]. We obtained proof for such a novel IL-2-binding molecule during examination of an NK-like cell line termed YT[3]. A Scatchard plot of binding to YT cells yielded a typical curvilinear plot indicative of high and intermediate-affinity binding. Inclusion of anti-Tac antibody in the assay eliminated the high-affinity binding component, but left the predominant intermediate-affinity ($K_d \sim 800$ pM) binding component intact. For convenience, we have termed this non-Tac IL-2 receptor "beta" (ß).

That ß was distinct from Tac protein was confirmed by crosslinking studies with ^{125}I-IL-2[3]. Covalent attachment of IL-2 to low-affinity Tac receptors yielded a 70,000 m.w. complex on SDS gels while crosslinking to the ß receptors on unstimulated YT cells yielded a doublet at 83 and 90,000 m.w. By inference, the size of the ß protein(s) was thus 70-75,000 m.w. Several other laboratories have independently reached similar conclusions with regard to the ß protein(s)[4-6]. The source of the size heterogeneity for ß-IL-2 complexes on SDS gels is still under investigation. Treatment of the complexes with glycosidases reduced their size by 15-20%, but did not totally eliminate the heterogeneity[3]. Thus, intermediate-affinity type II receptors may consist of two distinct proteins, although variable posttranslational modification or partial proteolytic degradation also remain likely causes of the differences in electrophoretic mobility.

ß receptors occur on several different lymphocyte subpopulations in the apparent absence of activation signals[18]. In contrast to the low-affinity Type I receptors, the ß chain by itself mediates rapid ligand internalization and certain cellular responses[19]. In particular, antibodies which selectively blocked ß-IL-2 interactions also inhibited the IL-2-dependent increase in the cytotoxic activity of NK cells, the IL-2-dependent induction of immunoglobulin secretion on a Tac-negative B cell line, and the IL-2-dependent upregulation of Tac protein on YT cells[20]. Thus, the ß chain is clearly a functional receptor for IL-2. It remains to be determined, however, whether additional non-Tac subunits exist which combine with the ß chain to form functional, intermediate-affinity receptors.

Type III Receptors - The Tac-IL-2-ß Complex

Due to their requirement for the Tac protein, high-affinity ($K_d \sim$ 5 to 20 pM) Type III IL-2 receptors generally occur only after cellular activation. Their abundance on such cells, however, is limited by the low level of expression of ß chains. Like the isolated ß chains, Type III receptors internalize ligand rapidly and mediate a variety of functional responses at low IL-2 concentrations.

Several lines of evidence indicate that it is the simultaneous binding of IL-2 by both the Tac and ß chains which provides the molecular basis for high-affinity binding sites. When YT cells were stimulated by forskolin, the number of Tac molecules on the cell surface and the number of high-affinity receptor sites increased dramatically[3]. At the same time, there was a parallel decrease in the original number of ß binding sites. Inclusion of anti-Tac in the assays for stimulated YT cells reversed these changes, eliminating the newly-formed high-affinity sites and restoring the original ß binding component. One explanation for these effects is that the induced Tac protein combined with ß to form high-affinity binding sites. Further supporting this concept, Dukovich et al.[18] found that transfection of a cell line containing ß protein with cDNA for the Tac subunit resulted in the conversion of some of the ß binding sites to a high-affinity state. Crosslinking studies also suggested the involvement of Tac and ß in high-affinity binding sites. Following binding to high-affinity sites on either a T lymphocytic cell line (HUT) or stimulated YT cells, IL-2 was crosslinked to the receptor in complexes (70,83 and 90,000 m.w.) characteristic of association with both the Tac (70,000 m.w. complex) and ß proteins (83-90,000 m.w.)[3]. As a final piece of evidence, we found that antibodies capable of selectively blocking the binding of IL-2 to Tac or to ß could each block ligand binding to high-affinity receptor sites, implying that both Tac and ß proteins were involved[3].

CONCLUDING REMARKS

Molecular characterization of the three forms of the IL-2 receptor has provided a clear explanation for both the differences in ligand affinity and the observations of cellular responses which were independent of the Tac receptor subunit. Looking to the future, cloning of the ß chain(s) will no doubt provide clues as to the initial enzymatic steps in signal transduction mediated by functional receptors. In addition, mutagenesis and crystallographic analyses of both the Tac and ß subunits will aid the design of IL-2 mimicks and antagonists which might facilitate therapeutic manipulation of the immune system.

REFERENCES

1. R. J. Robb, A. Munck, and K. A. Smith, T cell growth factor receptors: quantitation, specificity, and biological relevance, J. Exp. Med. 154:1455 (1981).
2. R. J. Robb, W. C. Greene, and C. M. Rusk, Low and high affinity cellular receptors for interleukin 2: implications for the level of Tac antigen, J. Exp. Med. 160:1126 (1984).
3. R. J. Robb, C. M. Rusk, J. Yodoi, and W. C. Greene, An interleukin 2 binding molecule distinct from the Tac protein: analysis of its role in formation of high-affinity receptors, Proc. Natl. Acad. Sci. USA 84:2002 (1987).
4. M. Sharon, R. D. Klausner, B. R. Cullen, R. Chizzonite, and W. J. Leonard, Novel interleukin 2 receptor subunit detected by crosslinking under high-affinity conditions, Science 234:859 (1980).
5. M. Tsudo, R. W. Kozak, C. K. Goldman, and T. A. Waldmann, Demonstration of a new non-Tac peptide that binds interleukin 2: a potential participant in a multichain interleukin-2 receptor complex, Proc. Natl. Acad. Sci USA 83:9694 (1986).
6. K. Teshigawara, H.-M. Wang, K. Kato, and K. A. Smith, Interleukin 2 high-affinity receptor expression requires two distinct binding proteins, J. Exp. Med. 165:223 (1987).
7. W. J. Leonard, J. M. Depper, T. Uchiyama, K. A. Smith, T. A. Waldmann, and W. C. Greene, A monoclonal antibody that appears to recognize the receptor for human T cell growth factor, Nature 300:267 (1982).
8. M. Hatakeyama, S. Minamoto, T. Uchiyama, R. R. Hardy, G. Yamada, and T. Taniguchi, Reconstitution of functional receptor for human interleukin-2 in mouse cells, Nature 318:467 (1985).
9. S. Kondo, A. Shimizu, M. Maeda, Y. Tagaya, J. Yodoi, and T. Honjo, Expression of functional human interleukin 2 receptor in mouse T cells by cDNA transfection, Nature 320:75 (1986).
10. S. Kondo, A. Shimizu, Y. Saito, M. Kinoshita, and T. Honjo, Molecular basis for two different affinity states of the interleukin 2 receptor: affinity conversion model, Proc. Natl. Acad. Sci. USA 83:9026 (1986).
11. R. J. Robb, Conversion of low-affinity interleukin 2 receptors to a high-affinity state following fusion of cell membranes, Proc. Natl. Acad. Sci. USA 83:3992 (1986).
12. M. Fujii, K. Sugamura, K. Sano, M. Nakai, K. Sugita, and Y. Hinuma, High-affinity receptor-mediated internalization and degradation of interleukin 2 in human T cells, J. Exp. Med. 163:550 (1986).
13. L.-M. Kuo, C. M. Rusk, and R. J. Robb, Structure-function relationships for the IL 2-receptor system II. Localization of an IL 2 binding site in high and low-affinity receptors, J. Immunol. 137:1544 (1986).
14. M. P. Neeper, L.-M Kuo, M. C. Kiefer, and R. J. Robb, Structure-function relationships for the IL 2-receptor system. III. Tac protein missing amino acids 102-173 (exon 4) is unable to bind IL 2. Detection of spliced protein after L cell transfection, J. Immunol. 138:3532 (1987).
15. C. M. Rusk, M. P. Neeper, L.-M. Kuo, R. M. Kutny and R. J. Robb, Structure-function relationships for the IL-2 receptor system. V. Structure-activity analysis of modified and truncated forms of the Tac receptor protein. Site-specific mutagenesis of cysteine residues, J. Immunol. in press.
16. J. R. Ortaldo, A. T. Mason, J. P. Gerard, L. E. Henderson, W. Farrar, R. F. Hopkins, R. B. Herberman, and H. Rabin, Effects of natural and recombinant IL-2 on regulation of IFN $_{3d}$ production and natural killer activity: lack of involvement of the Tac antigen for these immunoregulatory effects, J. Immunol. 133:779 (1984).
17. P. Ralph, G. Jeong, K., Welte, R. Mertelsmann, H. Rabin, L. E. Henderson, L. M. Souza, T. C. Boone, and R. J. Robb, Stimulation of immunoglobulin secretion in human B lymphocytes as a direct effect of high concentration of IL-2, J. Immunol. 133:2442 (1984).

18. M. Dukovich, Y. Wano, Le Thi Bich Thuy, P. Katz, B. R. Callen, J. H. Kerhl and W. C. Greene, A second human interleukin 2 binding protein that may be a component of high-affinity interleukin-2 receptors, Nature 327:518 (1987).
19. R. J. Robb, and W. C. Greene, Internalization of interleukin 2 is mediated by the beta chain of the high-affinity IL-2 receptor, J. Exp. Med. 165:1201 (1987).
20. R. J. Robb, Structure-function relationships for the interleukin 2 receptor. In: Molecular and Cellular Aspects of Inflammation G. Poste and S.T. Cooke, eds., Plenum Press, NY, pp. 97-122 (1988).

B LYMPHOCYTE DEVELOPMENT AND B CELL ACTIVATION

CELLULAR AND MOLECULAR REQUIREMENTS FOR B LYMPHOPOIESIS

Jeffrey M. Gimble, Shin-Ichi Hayashi, Carolynn E. Pietrangeli,
Grace Lee, and Paul W. Kincade

Oklahoma Medical Research Foundation
825 N.E. 13th Street
Oklahoma City, OK 73104

INTRODUCTION

At certain levels, the subject of B lymphocyte differentiation is no longer a mystery. Molecular biological approaches have helped explain the generation of antibody diversity as well as the mechanisms of immunoglobulin gene regulation[1]. Nevertheless, some areas still remain fruitful for investigation. The bone marrow is the bursal equivalent in adult mammals. This is the site where B lymphocyte differentiation begins from a putatitive multipotent hemopoietic stem cell. With cells of at least eight different hematopoeitic lineages all confined within a calcified matrix, attempts to address the bone marrow as an organ system have been difficult at best. However, recent advances in methodology have provided an experimental system for in vitro modeling of the bone marrow microenvironment. This paper will focus on the recently characterized "stromal" cells which support B lymphopoiesis and their potential relevance to physiologic and pathologic processes.

STROMAL CELLS

The concept of a bone marrow microenvironment supporting mammalian B lymphopoiesis can be dated to early physiologic and anatomic studies following the description of the avian bursa of Fabricius as the site of B lymphocyte development. Studies with lethally irradiated mice demonstrated that both lympho- and hematopoiesis could be reconsitituted by the intravenous administration of small numbers of bone marrow derived cells[2]. These and other studies proved that the bone marrow contained the lymphoid and hematologic stem cells[3,4]. Ultrastructural analysis of the bone marrow by scanning and transmission electron microscopy revealed the bone marrow to be a complex organ with localized compartments of differentiation[5,6]. Lymphopoiesis, myelopoiesis and erythropoiesis all occurred within a meshwork of adventitial reticular cells and vascular sinusoids[6]; this network of supporting cells became known as "stroma" [6].

The studies of Dexter et al. examining in vitro the growth of myeloid cells in cultured bone marrow specimens underlies the development of long term bone marrow cultures[7-9]. These workers observed that in the presence of horse serum and dexamethasone at 33 degree C, an adherent cell layer was established consisting of phagocytic mononuclear cells, epithelial-like cells and "giant fat" cells[9]. These adherent cells provided a nurturing environment for both pluripotent stem cells and committed granulocytic precursors over a period of months. While the number of stromal cells remained constant, the non-adherent granulocytes underwent many population doublings[9].

Whitlock and Witte exploited this system to investigate B lymphocyte differentiation in vitro[10,11]. Their culture system differed from that of Dexter; low concentrations of fetal calf serum supplemented with 2-mercaptoethanol replaced horse serum, dexamethasone was omitted and the temperature was raised to 37 degrees C[10,11]. They first observed that the adherent cell layer of cultured murine bone marrow cells proliferated, reaching confluency. At the same time, the number of non-adherent cells declined. However, after 3 to 4 weeks of culture, early stages of B lymphocytes made up a large proportion of the developing non-adherent cell population. In more extended cultures, mature lymphocytes expressing surface IgM and IgD were also conspicuous. These cultures, which could be successfully maintained for 6 months, were termed Long Term Bone Marrow Cultures (LTBMC)[10,11]. Presumably, the differing environments of the Dexter and Whitlock/Witte culture conditions either favor the committment of a pluripotent stem cell to a specific pathway or promote the proliferation of only a single lineage's committed precursor. However, the two culture systems are not mutually exclusive; the B lymphoid precursor cells will survive under Dexter conditions. "Switch" cultures in which bone marrow is grown under first Dexter and then Whitlock/Witte conditions will sequentially support granulopoiesis and lymphopoiesis[12-15]. The same adherent cell layer is capable of supporting both cell lineages.

The LTBMC system provides an exciting new approach to investigating the phenomenon of B lymphopoiesis in the bone marrow microenvironment. Nevertheless, caution must be exercised in evaluating these experiments. For example, in LTBMC experiments performed with bone marrow from Severe Combined Immunodeficient Disease (SCID) mice, an apparently normal proliferation of B lymphocytes occurs in culture despite the fact that peripheral B and T lymphocytes are almost undetectable in these animals in vivo[16]. However, the cultured SCID B lymphocytes themselves are abnormal with a high percentage of non-productive IgH gene rearrangements. This indicates that the normal "quality control" mechanisms functioning in vivo are not reproduced in the in vitro culture system[16]. Therefore, many of the cultured lymphocytes in LTBMC are defective and possibly pre-malignant[16]. Likewise, in vitro studies on motheaten (me) mouse bone marrow are consistent with the presence of an inhibitory factor or a direct interaction blocking lympho-hemopoiesis. This activity must be counter-regulated in the motheaten mouse as evidenced by the comparatively normal number of peripheral B lymphocytes[17]. Finally, in CBA/N strain mice, the accelerated outgrowth of lymphocytes in LTBMC is inconsistent with in vivo observations of B lineage population dynamics[18,19]. Together, these findings underline the fact that an in vitro model is only an approximation of the intact organ system.

Cells in the adherent layer of LTBMC consist of two morphologically distinct subpopulations[20,21]. Greater than 50% of the cells exhibit macrophage-like properties. They contain non-specific esterases and acid phosphatase and will phagocytize foreign material[20,21]. A second group of cells have been termed "stromal" cells. These are large, diffusely spreading cells which have been compared to endothelial or fibroblast cells[20,21]. In uncloned bone marrow cultures, clusters of developing lymphocytes are observed binding tightly to one stromal cell but not to its neighbors. This interaction is sufficiently strong to withstand the pull of gravity. In LTBMC established for a month in hanging drop cultures, viable lymphocytes can still be observed bound to the stromal cell layer (unpublished observations). This type of data suggests that a unique cell population exists within the bone marrow capable of supporting B lymphopoiesis. Attempts at deriving immortal stromal cell lines from murine tissues have been successful in several laboratories[13,14,15,22]. In our own lab,permanent stromal cell clones were established from whole organs treated with 5-Fluorouracil (5-FU). This drug eliminates a variety of hemopoietic cells and enriches for the outgrowth of an adherent cell layer consisting of macrophages and stromal cells. Repeated passage of those cells surviving 5-FU treatment resulted in the isolation of purified stromal cell lines. These stromal cell lines were tested for their ability to support B lymphocyte growth using a methyl cellulose cloning assay. A stromal cell dependent, B lymphocyte clone was plated onto the various stromal cell lines. Those stromal cell clones capable of supporting division in 20-80% of the plated B lymphocytes were termed "support" stromal cells to distinguish them from the "non-support" stromal cell clones. Morphologically, the two groups of stromal cell clones appeared the same. A number of support and non-support stromal cell clones were derived from bone marrow and spleen (Pietrangeli, MS in preparation).

CHARACTERIZATION OF STROMAL CELLS

Factor Production

While it is tempting to postulate that a single "poietin" is responsible for the differentiation of the B lymphocyte lineage, the existing data implies that this is an oversimplification. B cell precursors posssess functional receptors for IL-1, IFN-gamma, TGF-Rb, IL-4 as well as factors produced by autoimmune mice and patients with cyclic neutropenia.[1] Receptors for IL-2 and IL-3 have also been reported[23]. The importance of individual factors may change with the developmental state of B lymphocytes. For example, TGF-Rb inhibits the induction of kappa light chain gene expression in pre-B cells by known stimuli but does not block ongoing kappa synthesis in B cells[24]. Some variants of the 70Z/3 pre-B cell line are inducible for kappa expression by both LPS and IFN-gamma. However, the differential sensitivity to inhibition by TGF-Rb suggests that expression and regulation of the same gene may result from alternate transmembrane pathways[24].

Work is in progress in a number of labs to determine the factors produced by stromal cells which are required for B lymphocyte support. Growth factors and lymphokines can be assayed functionally, measuring the effect of conditioned media on an indicator cell line. Experiments have been performed supplementing LTBMC and cloned stromal cell lines with IL-4, also known as B-cell stimulatory factor-1[25]. In LTBMC, IL-4 inhibited the generation of pre-B cells. Likewise, it inhibited the proliferation of a stromal cell dependent pre-B cell line, blocking the nurturing effect of a supporting stromal cell[25]. However, the growth factors made by stromal cells may be labile and only present at low concentrations. Moreover, because of the intimate contact between stromal cells and developing lymphocytes, growth factors may be expressed on the surface of stromal cells in high local concentrations, rather than released and diluted in the microenvironment. This line of enquiry will most likely be pursued with molecular biological techniques. The high sensitivity of mRNA detection assays together with subtractive cloning approaches should establish what factors the stromal cells can make. With this information, it may be possible to determine which combination and concentration of factors is necessary to create a B lymphocyte supportive environment.

Cell Surface Markers

The expression of various cell surface markers on both uncloned LTBMC and cloned support and non-support stromal cell lines has been studied using monoclonal antibodies. So far, two general conclusions can be drawn from this work. First, no single marker differentiates support from non-support stromal cell clones. Second, in a number of cases, markers are expressed on cloned stromal cells which were absent on the stromal cells in the initial cultures.

In primary LTBMC cells, the hemopoietic cell antigen recognized by the monoclonal antibody M 1/69 is not expressed. This is a heat stable antigen expressed on erythrocytes, B lymphocytes, monocytes and granulocytes[26,27]. However, it was present on three out of 5 stromal cell clones tested. Likewise, all of the stromal cell clones are Thy-1 and Mac-3 positive while cells in the primary cultures are negative. There are several explanations for this difference. In continuous culture, stromal cells may adapt by taking on new features. Alternatively, the cloning process may have selected for a small sub-population of the primary culture whose surface properties went undetected. Finally, the development of a homogeneous cell population may have resulted in a autocrine phenomenon. Stromal cells may produce factors which, at high enough concentrations and in the absence of antagonists produced by other cell types, induce the expression of particular surface proteins.

Additional surface proteins expressed by stromal cells include Qa-2 and N-CAM. These proteins, together with Thy-1, can be linked to the cell membrane through phosphatidyl inositol (PI)[28-31]. The enzyme PI-PLC (phospholipase C) specifically cleaves the phosphatidyl inositol bond linking such proteins to the membrane[28,29]. Treatment of LTBMC with PI-PLC detaches up to 60% of the adherent lymphocytes suggesting that some of these proteins may be intermediates in the intimate lymphocyte/stromal cell adhesion[21]. N-CAM is one candidate for this role. In neural and muscle cells, several isoforms of the N-CAM protein derive from a single gene through a mechanism of alternative splicing[32-37]. This is detected by both multiple sized proteins on Western blots and multiple sized mRNAs on Northern blots. Western blot analysis of N-CAM proteins in stromal cells reveals one major (155 kd) and two minor isoforms[38]. Likewise, Northern blot analysis of stromal cell mRNA with an N-CAM probe detects three different sized transcripts at similar steady state levels (unpublished observation). The isoform pattern of N-CAM in stromal cells is not identical to that of either neural or muscle cells. N-CAM is postulated to play a role in cell adhesion through a homophilic interaction, i.e., one N-CAM molecule binding to another. One isoform of the protein in neural cells possesses an intracellular domain capable of interacting with actin, thus linking the membrane surface to the cytoskeleton[39]. Work is currently in progress cloning the N-CAM gene from a stromal cell cDNA library. Additional characterization of this protein in stromal cells may determine its role in supporting B lymphopoiesis.

The expression of surface proteins may potentially indicate the lineage derivation of the stromal cell lines. Three of the proteins, Qa-2, Thy -1 and N-CAM, are members of the immunoglobulin gene superfamily[40,41]. While Thy - 1 was originally defined as a T lymphocyte marker, both of Thy-1 and N-CAM are expressed on neuronal cells. In addition, stromal cells are positive for the macrophage markers, Mac-2 and Mac-3, but lack Mac-1 and F4/80. Spleen derived stromal cell clones take up acetylated LDL, consistent with a macrophage or endothelial cell origin, while their bone marrow derived counterparts do not. Of equal importance are those markers which are absent from stromal cells. Proteins commonly expressed on hemopoietic cells like Ly-5/CD45 (the common leukocyte antigen), members of the LFA-1 family, Class II antigens and Lpg-100 are not detected by monoclonal antibodies on LTBMC and cloned stromal cells([21] and Pietrangeli, MS in preparation). For these reasons, the lineage derivation of stromal cells remains uncertain. Further characterization with both monoclonal antibodies and mRNA probes is in progress to clarify their origin. Ultimately, it may be possible to determine the location of stromal cells on an embryological "fate map".

FUTURE APPLICATIONS OF STROMAL CELL RESEARCH

Normal Physiology

The physiologic process committing a pluripotent stem cell to the B lymphocyte lineage is unknown compared with our understanding of the events controlling later stages in B lymphocyte development. Molecular biology has recently provided the tools to explain the intricacies of gene rearrangement and to uncover the existence of immunoglobulin enhancers and repressors[42-47]. However, without the availability of cloned B lymphocytes representing different stages of maturation, these questions would not have been accessible to molecular biological expertise. At the present time, the development of stromal cell clones opens new experimental avenues. With these cells, it will be possible to expand and study, both at the cellular and molecular level, the earliest B lymphocyte precursors. Moreover, investigators may now be able to design direct experiments to determine the events which irreversibly commit a cell to the B lineage. Possibly, even the elusive "pluripotent" stem cell will be identified. Work has already begun along these lines. Various laboratories have followed the progressive rearrangement of immunoglobulin heavy chain genes in B lymphocytes supported in vitro by stromal cells[11,22,48]. As our understanding of stromal cells expands, it can be applied to the other hematologic cell lineages. Similar stromal cell clones supporting megakaryocytes, eosinophils and basophils may be developed as a consequence of long term culture studies in the lymphoid and myeloid lineages.

Pathophysiology

In recent years, there has been increasing utilization of bone marrow transplantation in conjunction with chemotherapy as a therapeutic modality for malignancy, aplastic anemia and SCIDs. Although the number of patients undergoing such treatment remains low, it represents a significant portion of the nation's medical expense. For this reason alone, it is obvious that any additional information about the bone marrow microenvironment will be valuable to future clinical practice. An increased analysis of stromal cells may improve the rate of bone marrow regeneration post-transplant, possibly through the addition of specific growth factors to the therapeutic regimen. Likewise, improved methods for handling bone marrow for transplant may result.

In addition, with the rapid advancements in recombinant DNA technology, the prospect of gene therapy may become a reality[49]. In specific disorders characterized by a defective or absent gene, vectors such as retroviruses will be designed to carry the missing gene into affected individuals. Bone marrow transplantation has been suggested as one possible route for such treatment. This methodology would require that the gene be introduced into a long lived cell line where it would not only be expressed but be delivered to its normal target tissue at effective levels. As more is learned about the lifespan of stromal cells and how they interact with developing hematologic cells, this cell lineage may possess important advantages as a target for this treatment. These speculations point out a more immediate practical consideration; at the present time, the reported stromal cell clones have been derived from murine systems. Investigators should begin to develop lines from human tissues.

REFERENCES

1. P.W. Kincade, Experimental models for understanding B lymphocyte formation, Adv.Immunol. 41:181 (1987).
2. S. Abramson, R.G. Miller and R.A. Phillips, The identification in adult bone marrow of pluripotent and restricted stem cells of the myeloid and lymphoid systems, J.Exp.Med. 145:1567 (1977).
3. J.J. Trentin, Determination of bone marrow stem cell differentiation by stromal hemopoietic inductive microenvironments (HIM), Am.J.Pathol. 65:621 (1971).
4. J.L. Curry and J.J. Trentin, Hemopoietic spleen colony studies. I. Growth and differentiation, Dev.Biol. 15:395 (1967).
5. L. Weiss, Hematopoietic microenvironment of the bone marrow: An ultrastructural study of the stroma in rats, Anat.Rec. 186:161 (1976).
6. L. Weiss and H. Sakai, The hematopoietic stroma, Am.J.Anat. 170:447 (1984).
7. T.D. Allen and T.M. Dexter, Cellular interrelationships during in vitro granulopoiesis, Differentiation 6:192 (1976).
8. T.M. Dexter and L.G. Lajtha, Proliferation of hematopoietic stem cells in vitro, Br.J.Haematol. 28:525 (1974).
9. T.M. Dexter, T.D. Allen and L.G. Lajtha, Conditions controlling the proliferation of haemopoietic stem cells in vitro, J.Cell Physiol. 91:335 (1977).
10. C.A. Whitlock, D. Robertson and O.N. Witte, Murine B cell lymphopoiesis in long-term culture, J.Immunol.Methods 67:353 (1984).
11. C. Whitlock, K. Denis, D. Robertson and O. Witte, In vitro analysis of murine B-cell development, Ann.Rev.Immunol. 3:213 (1985).
12. K. Dorshkind, In vitro differentiation of B lymphocytes from primitive hemopoietic precursors present in long-term bone marrow cultures, J.Immunol. 136:422 (1986).
13. A. Johnson and K. Dorshkind, Stromal cells in myeloid and lymphoid long-term bone marrow cultures can support multiple hemopoietic lineages and modulate their production of hemopoietic growth factors, Blood 68:1348 (1986).
14. L.S. Collins and K. Dorshkind, A stromal cell line from myeloid long-term bone marrow cultures can support myelopoiesis and B lymphopoiesis, J.Immunol. 138:1082 (1987).
15. P. Hunt, D. Robertson, D. Weiss, D. Rennick, F. Lee and O.N. Witte, A single bone marrow-derived stromal cell type supports the in vitro growth of early lymphoid and myeloid cells, Cell 48:997 (1987).

16. P.L. Witte, P.D. Burrows, P.W. Kincade and M.D. Cooper, Characterization of B lymphocyte lineage progenitor cells from mice with severe combined immune deficiency disease (SCID) made possible by long term culture, J.Immunol. 138:2698 (1987).
17. S-I. Hayashi, P.L. Witte, L.D. Shultz and P.W. Kincade, Lymphohemopoiesis in culture is prevented by interaction with adherent bone marrow cells from mutant viable motheaten mice, J. Immunol. (1988).(In Press)
18. S-I. Hayashi, P.L. Witte and P.W. Kincade, Studies of two genetically defective strains of mice in long term bone marrow culture, Fed.Proc. 46:1348 (1987).(Abstract)
19. G.K. Reid and D.G. Osmond, B lymphocyte production in the bone marrow of mice with X-linked immunodeficiency (xid), J.Immunol. 135:2299 (1985).
20. P.L. Witte, P.W. Kincade and V. Vetvicka, Interculture variation and evolution of B lineage lymphocytes in long-term bone marrow culture, Eur. J. Immunol. 16:779 (1986).
21. P.L. Witte, M. Robinson, A. Henley, M.G. Low, D.L. Stiers, S. Perkins, R.A. Fleischman and P.W. Kincade, Relationships between B-lineage lymphocytes and stromal cells in long term bone marrow cultures, Eur.J.Immunol. 17:1473 (1987).
22. C.A. Whitlock, G.F. Tidmarsh, C. Muller-Sieburg and I.L. Weissman, Bone marrow stromal cell lines with lymphopoietic activity express high levels of a pre-B neoplasia-associated molecule, Cell 48:1009 (1987).
23. P. Sideras and R. Palacios, Bone marrow pro-T and pro-B lymphocyte clones express functional receptors for interleukin (IL) 3 and IL 4/BSF-1 and nonfunctional receptors for IL 2, Eur.J.Immunol. 17:217 (1987).
24. G. Lee, L.R. Ellingsworth, S. Gillis, R. Wall and P.W. Kincade, B transforming growth factors are potential regulators of B lymphopoiesis, J. Exp. Med. 166:1290 (1987).
25. D. Rennick, G. Yang, C. Muller-Sieburg, C. Smith, N. Arai, Y. Takabe and L. Gemmell, Interleukin 4 (B-cell stimulatory factor 1) can enhance or antagonize the factor-dependent growth of hemopoietic progenitor cells, Proc.Natl.Acad.Sci.USA 84:6889 (1987).
26. T. Springer, G. Galfre, D.S. Secher and C. Milstein, Monoclonal xenogeneic antibodies to murine cell surface antigens: Identification of novel leukocyte differentiation antigens, Eur.J.Immunol. 8:539 (1978).
27. T.A. Springer, Monoclonal antibody analysis of complex biological systems, J.Biol.Chem. 256:3833 (1981).
28. H-T. He, J. Barbet, J-C. Chaix and C. Goridis, Phosphatidylinositol is involved in the membrane attachment of NCAM-120, the smallest component of the neural cell adhesion molecule, EMBO 5:2489 (1986).
29. M.G. Low, Biochemistry of the glycosyl-phosphatidylinositol membrane protein anchors, Biochem.J. 244:1 (1987).
30. M.G. Low and A.R. Saltiel, Structural and functional roles of glycosyl-phosphatidylinositol in membranes, Science (1988).(In Press)
31. M.G. Low, J. Stiernberg, G.L. Waneck, R.A. Flavell and P.W. Kincade, Cell based heterogeneity in sensitivity of phosphatidylinositol linked membrane antigens to release by phospholipase C, (1988).(UnPub)
32. G.C. Owens, G.M. Edelman and B.A. Cunningham, Organization of the neural cell adhesion molecule (N-CAM) gene: Alternative exon usage as the basis for different membrane-associated domains, Proc.Natl.Acad.Sci.USA 84:294 (1987).
33. G. Gennarini, M-R. Hirsch, H-T. He, M. Hirn, J. Finne and C. Goridis, Differential expression of mouse neural cell adhesion molecule (N-CAM) mRNA species during brain development and in neural cell lines, J.Neuroscience 6:1983 (1986).
34. S.E. Moore, J. Thompson, V. Kirkness, J.G. Dickson and F.S. Walsh, Skeletal muscle neural cell adhesion molecule (N-CAM): Changes in protein and mRNA species during myogenesis of muscle cell lines, J. Cell Biol. 105:1377 (1987).
35. G. Dickson, H.J. Gower, C.H. Barton, H.M. Prentice, V.L. Elsom, S.E. Moore, R.D. Cox, C. Quinn, W. Putt and F.S. Walsh, Human muscle neural cell adhesion molecule (N-CAM): Identification of a muscle-specific sequence in the extracellular domain, Cell 50:1119 (1987).

36. C. Goridis, M. Hirn, M-J. Santoni, G. Gennarini, H. Deagostini-Bazin, B.R. Jordan, M. Kiefer and M. Steinmetz, Isolation of mouse N-CAM-related cDNA: detection and cloning using monoclonal antibodies, EMBO 4:631 (1985).
37. B.A. Murray, J.J. Hemperly, E.A. Prediger, G.M. Edelman and B.A. Cunningham, Alternatively spliced mRNAs code for different polypeptide chains of the chicken neural cell adhesion molecule (N-CAM), J. Cell Biol. 102:189 (1986).
38. P.S. Thomas, C.E. Pietrangeli, S-I. Hayashi, M. Schachner, C. Goridis, M.G. Low and P.W. Kincade, Demonstration of neural cell adhesion molecules on stromal cells which support lymphopoiesis, Leukemia (1988).(In Press)
39. B.A. Cunningham, J.J. Hemperly, B.A. Murray, E.A. Prediger, R. Brackenbury and G.M. Edelman, Neural cell adhesion molecule: structure, immunoglobulin-like domains, cell surface modulation, and alternative RNA splicing, Science 236:799 (1987).
40. L. Hood, M. Kronenberg and T. Hunkapiller, T cell antigen receptors and the immunoglobulin supergene family, Cell 40:225 (1985).
41. A.F. Williams, A year in the life of the immunoglobulin superfamily, Immunol. Today 8:298 (1987).
42. N. Hozumi and S. Tonegawa, Evidence for somatic rearrangement of immunoglobulin genes coding for variable and constant regions, Proc.Natl.Acad.Sci.USA 73:3628 (1976).
43. J.G. Seidman and P. Leder, The arrangement and rearrangement of antibody genes, Nature 276:790 (1978).
44. R. Grosschedl and D. Baltimore, Cell-type specificity of immunoglobulin gene expression is regulated by at least three DNA sequence elements, Cell 41:885 (1985).
45. L. Emorine, M. Kuehl, L. Weir, P. Leder and E.E. Max, A conserved sequence in the immunoglobulin J_K-C_K intron: possible enhancer element, Nature 304:447 (1983).
46. C. Queen and D. Baltimore, Immunoglobulin gene transcription is activated by downstream sequence elements, Cell 33:741 (1983).
47. C. Queen and J. Stafford, Fine mapping of an immunoglobulin gene activator, Mol. Cell. Biol. 4:1042 (1984).
48. K. Hirayosh, S-I. Nishikawa, T. Kina, M. Hatanaka, S. Habu, T. Nomura and Y. Katsura, Immunoglobulin heavy chain gene diversification in the long-term bone marrow culture of normal mice and mice with severe combined immunodeficiency, Eur.J.Immunol. 17:1051 (1987).
49. W.F. Anderson, Prospects for human gene therapy, Science 226:401 (1984).

TRANSCRIPTIONAL REGULATION OF IMMUNOGLOBULIN HEAVY CHAIN AND T-CELL RECEPTOR BETA CHAIN GENES

Skye McDougall*, Suzanne Eaton#, Craig L. Peterson# and Kathryn Calame+

*Laboratory of Biomedical and Environmental Science, UCLA, Los Angeles, CA 90024, #Department of Biochemistry and Biophysics UCSF, San Francisco, CA 94143; and + Department of Microbiology Columbia University College of Physicians and Surgeons, New York NY, 10032

INTRODUCTION

Transcription of immunoglobulin heavy chain (IgH) and T-cell receptor (TCR) beta chain genes is controlled in a tissue and developmental stage specific manner (Calame, 1985; Kronenberg et al., 1986). We are studying the DNA sequence elements and cellular proteins which regulate transcription of these two important gene families. Early in B-cell ontogeny IgH transcription is activated as a result of VDJ joining which brings a transcriptional enhancer within functional proximity of the rearranged promoter (Mercola et al., 1983; Banerji et al., 1983; Gilles et al., 1983; Neuberger, 1983; Wang and Calame, 1985). Similar gene rearrangements occur in the beta chain locus during T cell ontogeny; however, the elements responsible for regulation of TCR beta genes have not been well defined.

V_H promoters are subject to complex regulation during B cell development. They are expressed in an enhancer-independent fashion prior to VDJ joining and later in development become enhancer-dependent (Yancopoulos and Alt, 1985). V_H promoters as well as the IgH enhancer are responsible for restricting expression of heavy chain genes to B cells (Mason et al., 1985; Grosschedl and Baltimore, 1985). In earlier functional studies on the heavy chain promoter we identified four regions required for promoter activity in plasmacytomas (Eaton and Calame, 1987). We report here results of in vitro studies which demonstrate that multiple transcription factors, three of which have a tissue-specific distribution, bind to V_H promoters.

The mechanism by which the IgH enhancer interacts with IgH promoters to activate transcription is not understood. A combination of in vivo and in vitro studies has shown that the IgH enhancer binds a minimum of six different proteins which are required for its function (Peterson et al., 1986; Peterson and Calame, 1987; Schlokat et al., 1986; Sen and Baltimore, 1986; Ephrussi et al., 1985; Weinberger et al., 1986). We have purified one of these proteins, uEBP-E, to homogeneity and demonstrate that it also binds with high affinity to IgH promoters.

By analogy to Ig regulation, it is reasonable to expect that an enhancer may be located 5' of one or both TCR beta constant region gene segments which could activate transcription upon $V_BD_BJ_B$ joining. By comparing the transcription rates of unrearranged and rearranged V_B genes, we demonstrate that $V_BD_BJ_B$ joining does indeed activate V_B transcription, suggesting the presence of enhancer(s) in the beta chain locus. Using transient transfections we demonstrate: i) there is no enhancer detectable by our assay 5' of C_{B2}; ii) there is a stronger enhancer 7.5 kb 3' of C_{B2}.

ANALYSIS OF TRANSCRIPTION FACTORS WHICH BIND TO IgH PROMOTERS AND ENHANCER

In earlier studies, our laboratory identified four regions of the V1 heavy chain promoter that were required for normal levels of expression in B cells (Eaton and Calame, 1987). The conserved octanucleotide at -56 bp (numbering from the transcription start site) stimulates transcription at least 50 fold, a conserved heptamer at -70 bp stimulates transcription five fold, a region of purine/pyrimidine assymmetry is responsible for a two-fold increase in activity, and sequences between -251 and -125 bp have a two-fold effect on transcription. In more recent experiments, we have identified factors from nuclear extracts which bind to these functionally important sequences in vitro. Previously we have also demonstrated that there are eight protein binding sites within the mouse immunoglobulin heavy chain enhancer which are recognized by a minimum of six different cellular proteins (Peterson et al., 1986; Peterson and Calame, 1987). In vivo functional analyses have indicated that six of these protein binding sites are required for optimal enhancer activity (Tsao et al., 1988). Our current efforts are aimed at purifying and characterizing these promoter and enhancer proteins and understanding how they interact with DNA, with each other and with other proteins to establish stable transcription complexes at V_H promoters.

Nuclear Factor(s) Bind to the Conserved Heptamer

A conserved heptamer lies between 2 and 22 bp 5' of the octamer in different heavy chain V gene promoters. We examined partially purified nuclear extracts from murine plasmacytoma M603 using gel shift assays and orthophenanthroline/Cu (OP/Cu) chemical nuclease footprinting (Kuwabara and Sigman, 1987) to detect proteins which might bind to the heptamer. These experiments revealed nuclear factor(s), eluting from a Mono Q anion exchange column at 150 mM NaCl, which protected two regions: the heptamer and a sequence 30 bp 5' of the heptamer from chemical cleavage with OP/Cu. The OP/Cu footprint generated by this complex is shown in figure 1, panel III and summarized on the sequence below. Further purification will be necessary to determine whether this protection pattern results from binding of one or two proteins.

Fractions which elute from Mono Q columns at higher salt concentration contain a different heptamer-binding activity which generates a strong hypersensitive site around the heptamer region, but does not protect the additional upstream sequence. Its OP/Cu footprint is shown in figure 1., panel IV. Thus it seems likely that at least two different proteins may bind the heptamer.

The proximity of heptamer and octamer sequences suggests that the heptamer binding factors could affect the binding or activity of the octamer binding proteins. Positive interaction with the B-cell-specific octamer factor would be consistent with the increase in transcription observed when the heptamer is included in V_H gene promoters (Eaton and Calame, 1987; Ballard and Bothwell, 1986). Alternatively, heptamer factor may prevent the binding of ubiquitous octamer factors, preventing inappropriate activation of immunoglobulin genes in non-B cells. These possibilities can be tested by examining the interaction of purified heptamer binding protein with different octamer factors in vitro.

Tissue-Specific Proteins Bind 5' of the Heptamer/Octamer Region

Experiments in other laboratories have shown that lymphoid cells contain a unique form of octamer binding protein, which may be involved in the tissue specific activity of immunoglobulin genes (Landolfi et al., 1986; Staudt et al., 1986; Wirth et al., 1987). Functional analysis of the V1 heavy chain promoter demonstrated a positive transcription element located between -251 and -125 bp from the cap site (Eaton and Calame, 1987) and

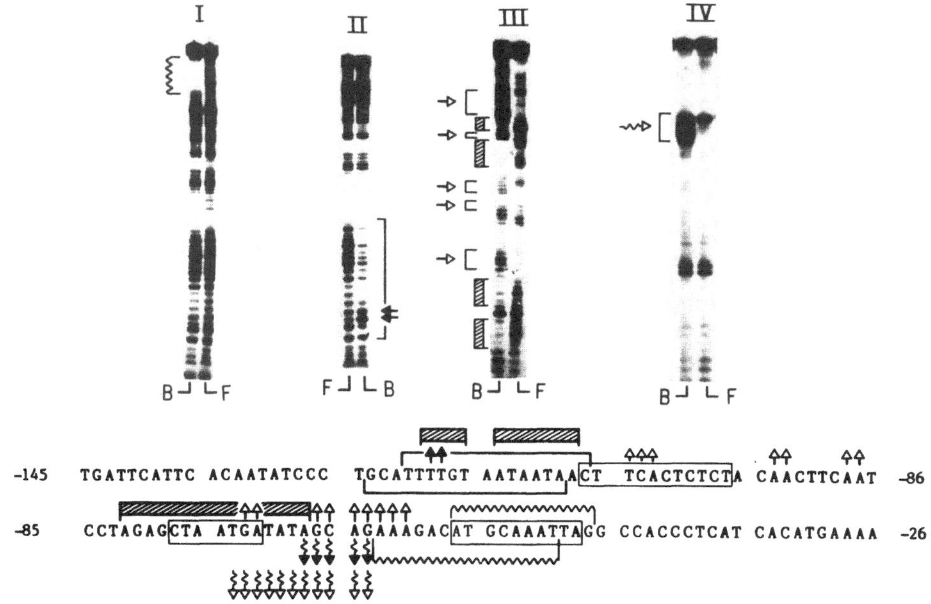

Figure 1. DNA/Protein Interactions in the V1 Promoter: -145 to -20.Panels I through IV depict OP/Cu footprinting experiments performed on the V1 promoter. The indicated DNA fragments were end labelled and incubated with either crude nuclear extracts or fractions eluted from an FPLC MonoQ anion exchange column. DNA/protein complexes derived from a subsequent preparative gel shift procedure were treated in the gel with the chemical nuclease orthophenanthroline and copper. Bound (B) and free (F) DNAs were eluted from the gel, extracted with phenol, and compared on 8% acrylamide 8M urea gels. The autoradiograms are shown. Regions of protection from cleavage are indicated next to the autoradiograms by bars (solid, open or hatched) and summarized on the sequence by bars of the same type. Regions of hypersensitivity are denoted by brackets and arrows (filled, solid, and wiggly) on the autoradiograms and summarized on the sequence by arrows of the same type. Panel I) probe: -145 to -32, protein: crude P3X nuclear extract. Panel II) probe: -57 to -145, protein: purified u-EBP-E. Panel III) probe: -145 to -32, protein: MonoQ 150MmMNaCl fraction. Panel IV) probe: -1 to -107, protein: MonoQ 350 mM NaCl fraction.

our in vitro protein binding studies suggest that this region may also be important in determining B-cell specificity of V_H promoters.

Gel shift assays performed with a probe containing the 5' region produce two DNA-protein complexes (LyA and LyB) when B cell extracts are used, and a single complex (F) when fibroblast extracts are examined (data not shown). The sequences involved in the formation of these complexes were examined by OP/Cu footprinting and methylation interference (figure 2). Panel I shows the OP/Cu footprint of complex LyA. The interaction which produces this complex results in both protection from and enhancement of OP/Cu mediated cleavage over a large region from -175 to -215 bp (summarized on the sequence below). Panel II depicts a methylation interference experiment performed on LyA. Those G's and A's which interfere with binding are indicated and summarized on the sequence below. The region defined by the LyA footprint contains a strong homology to the IgH enhancer D site (Peterson et al., 1986).

Complex F was observed only in gel shift experiments performed with fibroblast extracts and was not present in extracts from pre-B cell lines, a resting B cell line, or plasmacytomas. Methylation interference experiments showed that protection extends over a sequence centered at -150 (figure 2, panel III). This is consistent with its OP/Cu footprint (summarized in figure 2). We have preliminary evidence that protein present in the LyB complex binds a region which partially overlaps the fibroblast-specific protein binding site (data not shown).

Binding of proteins with a tissue-specific distribution to the region between -215 and -145 strongly suggest that this region is involved in restricting promoter activity to B cells. This restriction could be positive, negative, or both. The function of this upstream region may be redundant with that of the octamer in conferring B-cell-specificity. Further redundancy exists because both the heavy chain promoter and enhancer independently restrict expression to B cells. Perhaps multiple elements are necessary to assure strict restriction of immunoglobulin expression to B cells in vivo.

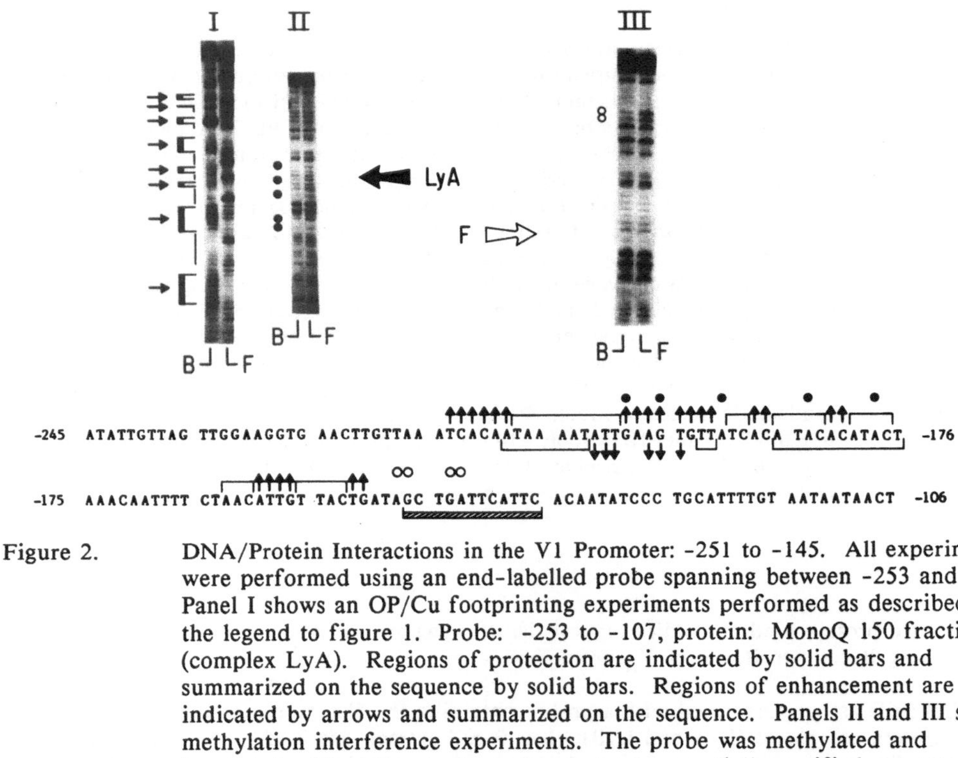

Figure 2. DNA/Protein Interactions in the V1 Promoter: -251 to -145. All experiments were performed using an end-labelled probe spanning between -253 and -107. Panel I shows an OP/Cu footprinting experiments performed as described in the legend to figure 1. Probe: -253 to -107, protein: MonoQ 150 fraction (complex LyA). Regions of protection are indicated by solid bars and summarized on the sequence by solid bars. Regions of enhancement are indicated by arrows and summarized on the sequence. Panels II and III show methylation interference experiments. The probe was methylated and incubated with either crude nuclear extract or partially purified extract as indicated. Bound (B) and free (F) probe were separated by electrophoresis on a 6% native acrylamide gel, eluted, and subjected to piperidine cleavage. Bound and free DNA were then compared on 8% acrylamide 8M urea gels. The autoradiograms are shown. Panel II) MonoQ fraction 19 (complex LyA). Panel III) L cell crude nuclear extract (complex F).

Transcription Factor uEBP-E Binds to Multiple Sites Including High Affinity Sites on Both the IgH Enhancer and IgH Promoters

A protein, uEBP-E, which binds to one of the functionally important regions of the IgH enhancer, site E, has been purified to apparent homogeneity by a combination of ion exchange and oligonucleotide affinity chromatography (Peterson et al., 1988). Once the purification of uEBP-E was complete, we wished to test whether this enhancer binding protein might bind to other sites within the IgH enhancer or to site(s) within an IgH promoter.

To test for other sites within the enhancer we used two DNA fragments for uEBP-E binding analyses. One of these fragments, a 220 bp RsaI-PstI fragment, contains the previously identified binding site E, and the second is a 190 bp PstI-HinfI fragment which contains sequences 3' to site E. To test for uEBP-E binding sites within a heavy chain promoter, we utilized a 110 bp DdeI-BamH1 fragment of the V1 promoter (Eaton and Calame, 1987). Figure 3 shows the results of a binding titration of purified uEBP-E on these three DNA probes and demonstrates that uEBP-E binds to another site on the IgH enhancer and to a site on the V1 promoter. In further studies, we find that uEBP-E also binds to another heavy chain promoter, 17.2.25, the Ig kappa enhancer, polyoma virus enhancer, and, with lower affinity to the Herpes virus tk promoter (data not shown). No binding was observed to the MOPC41 kappa promoter, however.

To map the uEBP-E binding sites on the IgH enhancer and the V1 promoter, we performed OP/Cu footprinting of the protein-DNA complexes (Peterson and Calame, 1987). In addition, we mapped the binding of uEBP-E to site E on the enhancer more precisely. These results are shown in figure 3. Site E was mapped between nucleotides 322 and 340 on the enhancer (panel D), and site E' is located 150 bp 3' of site E at position 467 to 485 (panel E). Within the V1 promoter, the uEBP-E site was mapped between -107 and -126bp with respect to the start site for transcription (panel F). This binding site is directly adjacent to the conserved pyrimidine element which is known from deletional analyses to be required for promoter function in vivo.

We wished to determine the binding affinity of uEBP-E for the two enhancer and V1 promoter sites. We used gel shift assays to obtain a saturation curve for uEBP-E binding to IgH enhancer site E. Scatchard analysis of the binding of uEBP-E to site E yielded an apparent equilibrium dissociation constant of 0.29 nM (data not shown). Knowing the equilibrium binding constant for site E, the binding constants for the two new sites could be determined relative to site E by comparing the amount of uEBP-E that is needed to bind 50% of each of the three probes. These experiments reveal that the site within the V1 promoter binds uEBP-E 1.2x better than site E on the enhancer, while the new enhancer binding site, which we have designated E', binds purified uEBP-E with 5.5x lower affinity than site E on the enhancer.

Deletions of high affinity site E for u-EBP-E in the enhancer reduce activity to 36% of wild type (Tsao et al., 1988), although mutation of site E' has no effect (Kiledjian et al., 1988). In the V1 promoter, u-EBP-E binds immediately 5' to the conserved strech of purine pyrimidine assymmetry (Eaton and Calame, 1987). This sequence lies in a region which progressive 5' deletion has shown to be necessary for full promoter activity (Eaton and Calame, 1987); however, the uEBP-E site has not yet been specifically mutated.

In addition to uEBP-E, octamer factors also bind to both IgH promoters and enhancer. Binding of u-EBP-E and octamer factors to both the enhancer and promoters may be involved in the synergistic interaction between these elements (Garcia et al., 1986). If uEBP-E and/or octamer factors have multiple DNA binding sites or dimerize, this would bring the enhancer and promoter into close proximity and would allow efficient interaction of proteins bound to the two elements. Alternatively, binding of uEBP-E and octamer factors to unrearranged promoters could be important for the enhancer-independent transcription of unrearranged V_H genes early in B-cell development (Yancopoulos and Alt, 1985).

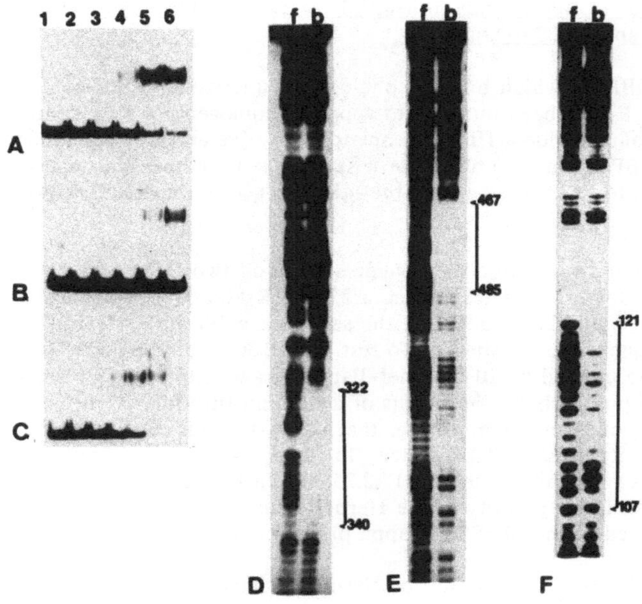

Figure 3. Binding analyses of affinity purified uEBP-E to sequences within the IgH enhancer and promoter elements. Panels A, B, and C represent gel retardation assays (Peterson and Calame, 1987) using affinity purified uEBP-E protein (see text). The DNA probe used for the assays in panel A was a RsaI-PstI enhancer fragment containing site E, assays in panel B used a PstI-HinfI enhancer fragment containing site E', and panel C assays used a probe containing the V1 heavy chain promoter. Numbered lanes above panel A indicate increasing amounts of purified uEBP-E used in the binding reactions for all three panels. Assays in lanes 1-6 utilized 0, 20, 40, 80, 120, and 200 pg of purified uEBP-E, respectively. Each assay contained the respective DNA probe at a concentration of 0.16 nM, and no nonspecific DNA was included. Panels D, E, and F represent ortho-phenanthroline/Cu chemical nuclease footprinting (Kuwabara and Sigman, 1987) of the protein- DNA complexes observed in panels A, B, and C, respectively. Lanes labeled f indicate the free DNA probe cleaved with the OP/Cu nuclease, and lanes labeled b indicate cleaved DNA purified from the protein DNA complex. Sequences protected from cleavage by the OP/Cu nuclease are indicated by brackets. The numbering system of Ephrussi et al., 1985 is used to indicate the position on the IgH enhancer, while the V1 promoter sequence is designated with respect to the start site of transcription.

IDENTIFICATION OF A TRANSCRIPTIONAL ENHANCER WHICH ACTIVATES V BETA TRANSCRIPTION

$V_2D_BJ_B$ Joining Activates TCR VB Gene Transcription

If, by analogy to Ig genes, a transcriptional enhancer were present in the the beta chain locus, we would expect that unrearranged V beta genes would not be transcribed but would be transcriptionally activated after VDJ joining. To test whether rearrangement is required to activate V_B transcription, we used run-on transcription in isolated nuclei. This assay quantitates polymerase loading on a particular region of DNA regardless of subsequent RNA processing or degradation and therefore reflects the transcription rate (Groudine et al., 1981). The results in table 1 show that in T cell hybridoma, BO4H.H.9.1, which expresses V_{B1} transcription of the unrearranged V_{B1} gene is undetectable although V_{B3} is transcribed. Similarly in the T cell line, SL3, which by northern analysis does not express V_{B3} (data not shown) there is only a low level of transcription from the unrearranged V_{B3} gene. In addition, the unrearranged V_{B3} gene was transcriptionally silent in plasmacytoma S107 and in NIH3T3 cells. The results of these experiments indicate: i) although there is a low level of transcription from unrearranged V_B genes in some T cells, rearrangement activates transcription and ii) unrearranged V_B gene segments are transcriptionally silent in non-T cells.

A Transcriptional Enhancer Is Located 7.5 kb 3' of the C_{B2} Gene Segment

The dependence of V_B transcription upon VDJ joining suggests that there may be enhancer(s) 5'of the C_B constant gene segments similar to these in the Ig heavy and kappa loci. We tested the region extending from D_{B1} through C_{B2} for the presence of enhancer activity by subcloning portions of this region 3' of the chloramphenicol acetyltransferase (CAT) gene in the vector pA10CAT2. This vector contains the SV40 early promoter directing transcription of the CAT gene but does not contain a functional SV40 enhancer (Gorman et al., 1982). The amount of CAT enzyme activity produced upon transfection of the T cell line EL4 with these constructs is a sensitive measure of the enhancer activity of a cloned sequence. In all cases, we used cotransfection with a plasmid expressing beta-galactosidase activity to correct for differences in transfection efficiency. The results are shown in Fig. 4. We find low, variable enhancer activity in the region between J_{B1} and C_{B1}. Further studies are underway to locate this activity more precisely; however, it is obvious that this enhancer could not activate transcription for genes which rearrange to D_{B2} since it would be deleted during rearrangement. A T-cell specific DNase I hypersensitive site has been reported in the J_{B2} to C_{B2} intron (Bier et al., 1985). Since enhancer regions are usually hypersensitive to DNase I, we tested this region with particular care; however, no enhancer activity was detectable in any of our constructs. Interestingly a region 7.5 kb 3' of C_{B2} showed strong activity, enhancing transcription of the SV40 promoter 4 to 9 fold over the enhancerless control (figure 4). Thus we conclude that while the general pattern of transcriptional activation by bringing an enhancer within functional proximity of a rearranged V gene promoter is conserved between Ig and TCR beta chain loci. Interestingly, the placement of the enhancer in the two loci is different (McDougall and Calame, 1988). It will be important to determine if the transcription factors required for activity of the TCR beta enhancer are similar or different from those required for Ig enhancers.

We also wanted to determine whether there is a synergistic interaction between a V_B promoter and the enhancer 3' of C_{B2} and what role, if any, each of these elements plays in the tissue specific expression of the TCR beta chain gene. A CAT vector containing 700 bp of the V_{B3} promoter was constructed. Either the beta enhancer or the SV40 enhancer was cloned into this vector 3' of the CAT gene. The beta enhancer was able to enhance transcription of the V_{B3} promoter 4 fold over the enhancerless control which is the same level of enhancement when the SV40 promoter was used. This lack of synergy between the beta promoter and enhancer differs from what is seen for the Ig heavy chain. Preliminary results of transfections into both B and L cells indicated that both the promoter and enhancer function only in T cells. This result for the enhancer is different from the Ig heavy chain enhancer, which is lymphoid specific.

Table 1. Radioactivity Obtained from Run-on Synthesis in Isolated Nuclei

		V_{B3}	V_{B1}	C_{B1}	DNA Probes B2M	GAPDH	VH14B	IGHE
Labeled RNA								
T Cells								
B04H.H.9.1	1	95	9	104	146	434	ND	ND
	2	30	0	31	91	203	ND	ND
SL3	1	11	ND	61	62	ND	0	ND
	2	27	ND	73	78	ND	0	ND
Non-T Cells								
NIH3T3	1	0	ND	0	69	55	0	ND
	2	0	ND	0	63	35	0	ND
S107	1	0	ND	ND	89	423	0	381

Each number represents the average radioactivity on duplicate dot filters, as determined by scintillation counting. The cpm have been corrected for the plasmid background and normalized for the length of the probe. The DNA probes were hybridized with 20-100x10 cpm of labeled RNA. The DNA probes are the following: V_{B1} and V_{B3} are V beta genes, C_{B1} is a beta chain C gene, B2M is B2-microglobulin, VH14B is a heavy chain V gene, IGHE is the heavy chain enhancer, GAPDH is the rat glyceraldhyde-3-phosphate dehydrogenase gene. B2M and GAPDH were simply used as internal controls for the assay. In the T and B cells where DNA rearranges the presence of the V_{B3} and V_{B1} genes was confirmed by probing genomic DNA with the V_{B1} and V_{B3} probes.

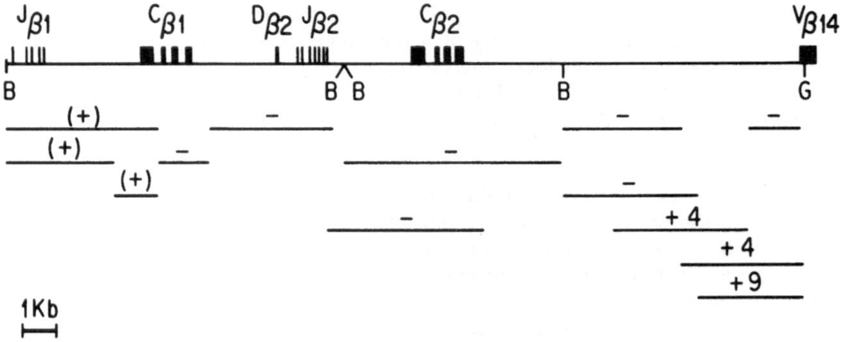

Figure 4. Analysis of the beta chain locus for a transcriptional enhancer. Restriction fragments were cloned into pA10CAT2. The constructs were transiently transfected by electroporation (Potter et al., 1984) into the T cell line, EL4, and enhancer activity was assayed for by measuring CAT activity. In all experiments a plasmid expressing beta-galactosidase was cotransfected to normalize for transfection efficiency. +4 and +9 indicates the fold enhancement of the construct over the enhancerless control, "-" indicates no enhancement and "(+)" denotes weak but unquantitated activity. B is BamH1 and G is Bgl1.

SUMMARY

We have identified factors that bind to functionally important regions in IgH chain promoters and enhancer. One promoter factors is identical to u-EBP-E, an enhancer binding protein. Several promoter-binding proteins are present preferentially in either B cells or fibroblasts although most enhancer-binding proteins have a ubiquitous distribution. Additional characterization of these factors will further our understanding of the mechanisms by which IgH promoters and enhancers interact to achieve B-cell restricted and developmental stage-specific expression of IgH genes. The identification of a TCR beta chain enhancer will allow us to pursue similar questions with respect to the regulated expression this locus.

REFERENCES

Ballard, D. and Bothwell, A., 1986, Mutational analysis of the immunoglobulin heavy chain promoter region, Proc. Natl. Acad. Sci. USA, 83:9626.

Banerji, J., Olson, L., and Schaffner, W., 1983, A lynphocyte-specific cellular enhancer is located downstream of the joining region in immunoglobulin heavy chain genes, Cell, 33:729.

Bier, N., Hashimoto, Y., Greene, M., and Maxam, A., 1985, Active T-cell receptor genes have intron deoxyribonuclease hypersensitive sites, Science, 229:528.

Calame, K., 1985, Mechanisms that regulate immunoglobulin gene expression, Ann. Rev. Immunol., 3:159.

Eaton, S., and Calame, K., 1987, Multiple DNA sequence elements are necessary for the function of an immunoglobulin heavy chain promoter, Proc. Natl. Acad. Sci. USA, 84:7634.

Ephrussi, A., Church, G., Tonegawa, S., and Gilbert, W., 1985, B lineage-specific interactions of an immunoglobulin enhancer with cellular factors in vivo, Science, 227:134.

Garcia, J., Thuy, L., Stafford, J., and Queen, C., 1986, Synergism between immunoglobulin enhancers and promoters, Nature, 322:383.

Gillies, S., Morrison, S., Oi, V., and Tonegawa, S., 1983, A tissue-specific transcription enhancer element is located in the major intron of a rearranged immunoglobulin heavy chain gene, Cell, 33:717.

Gorman, C., Moffat, L., and Howard, B., 1982, Recombinant genomes which express chloramphenicol acetyltransferase in mammalian cells, Mol. Cell. Biol, 2:1044.

Grosschedl, R., and Baltimore, D., 1985, Cell-type specificity of immunoglobulin gene expression is regulated by at least three DNA elements, Cell, 41:885.

Groudine, M., Peretz, M., and Weintraub, H., 1981, Transcriptional regulation of hemoglobin switching in chicken embryos, Mol. Cell. Biol., 3:281.

Kiledjian, M., Su, L., and Kadesch, T., 1988, Identification and characterization of two functional domains within the murine heavy chain enhancer, Mol. Cell. Biol., 8:145.

Kronenberg, M., Siu, G., Hood, L., and Shastri, N., 1986, The molecular genetics of the T-cell antigen receptor and T-cell antigen recognition, Ann. Rev. Immunol., 4:529.

Kuwabara, M., and Sigman, D., 1987, Footprinting DNA-protein complexes in situ following gel retardation assays using 1,10-phenanthroline-copper ion: Escherichia coli RNA polynerase-lac promoter complexes, Biochemistry, 26:7234.

Landolfi, N., Capra, J., and Tucker, P., 1986, Interaction of cell-type-specific nuclear proteins with immunoglobulin promoter sequences, Nature, 323:548.

Mason, J., Williams, G., and Neuberger, M., 1985, Transcriptional cell type specificity is conferred by an immunoglobulin Vh gene promoter that includes a functional consensus sequence, Cell, 41:479.

McDougall, S., and Calame, K., 1988, A transcriptional enhancer 3' of Cß2 in the T cell receptor B locus, Sci 241:205.

Mercola, M., Wang, X., Olsen, J., and Calame, K., 1983, Transcriptional enhancer elements in the mouse immunoglobulin heavy chain locus, Science, 221:663.

Neuberger, M., 1983, Expression and regulation of immunoglobulin heavy chain gene transfected into lymphoid cells, EMBO J., 2:1373.

Peterson, C., Orth, K., and Calame, K., 1986, Binding in vitro of multiple cellular proteins to immunoglobulin heavy-chain enhancer DNA, Mol. Cell. Biol., 6:4168.
Peterson, C., and Calame, K., 1987, Complex protein binding within the mouse immunoglobulin heavy-chain enhancer, Mol. Cell. Biol., 7:4194.
Peterson, C., Eaton, S., and Calame, K., 1988, Purified uEBP-E binds to immunoglobulin enhancers and promotors, Mol. Cell. Biol., in press.
Potter, H., Weir, L., and Leder, P., 1984, Enhancer-dependent expression of human K immunoglobulin genes introduced into mouse pre-B lymphocytes by electroporation, Proc. Natl. Acad. Sci. USA, 81:7161.
Royer, H., and Reinherz, E., 1987, Multiple nuclear proteins bind upstream sequences in the promoter region of a T-cell receptor B-chain variable-region gene: evidence for tissue specificity, Proc. Natl. Acad. Sci.USA.,84:232.
Schlokat, U., Bohmann, D., Scholer, H., and Gruss, P., 1986, Nuclear factors binding specific sequences within the immunoglobulin enhancer interact differentially with other enhancer elements, EMBO J., 5:3251.
Sen, R., and Baltimore, D., 1986, Multiple nuclear factors interact with the immunoglobulin enhancer sequences, Cell, 46:705.
Staudt, L., Singh, H., Sen, R., Wirth, T., Sharp, P., and Baltimore, D., 1986, A lymphoid-specific protein binding to the octamer motif of immunoglobulin genes, Nature, 323:640.
Tsao, B., Wang, X., Peterson, C., and Calame, K., 1988, In vivo functional analysis of in vitro protein binding sites in the immunoglobulin heavy chain enhancer, Submitted.
Weinberger, J., Baltimore, D., and Sharp, P., 1986, Distinct factors bind to apparently homologous sequences in the immunoglobulin heavy-chain enhancer, Nature, 322:846.
Wang, X., and Calame, K., 1985, The endogenous immunoglobulin heavy chain enhancer can activate tandem VH promoters separated by a large distance, Cell, 43:659.
Wirth, T., Staudt, T., and Baltimore, D., 1987, An octamer oligonucleotide upstream of a TATA motif is sufficient for lymphoid-specific promoter activity, Nature, 329:174
Yancopoulos, G., and Alt, F., 1985, Developmentally controlled and tissue specific expression of unrearranged VH gene segments, Cell, 40:271.

PRECURSOR B LYMPHOCYTES - SPECIFIC MONOCLONAL ANTIBODIES AND GENES

Fritz Melchers, Steven R. Bauer, Christoph Berger,
Hajime Karasuyama, Akira Kudo, Antonius Rolink,
Nobuo Sakaguchi, Andreas Strasser, and Philipp Thalmann

Basel Institute for Immunology
Basel
Switzerland

INTRODUCTION

The pool of mature, surface immunoglobulin (Ig) positive, antigen-sensitive B cells of a mouse has been estimated to contain 5 x 10^8 to 10^9 cells (Osmond 1986). Development from pluripotent stem cells and committed progenitors generates daily some 5 x 10^7 cells, of which 3 x 10^6 enter the pool of mature B cells. The same number of mature B cells must consequently die daily to keep the pool at a constant size. The immediate precursors of the mature B cells, called pre B cells, can be identified to be at various stages of their development by the genomic context in which their Ig gene loci are found. Thus, rearrangement of a D_H to a J_H seqment on the Ig heavy (H) chain locus precedes that of V_H to D_HJ_H. This, in turn, is followed by rearrangements of the Igκ light (L) chain and, finally, of the λ L chain locus (Tonegawa, 1983). No more than five divisions are estimated to occur from the earliest (i.e. at the time of D_H to J_H rearrangement) to the latest (i.e. at the time of surface Ig expression) state of their B lineage development in either fetal liver during embryogenesis or in bone marrow throughout adult life. The daily generation of 5 x 10^7 cells must, therefore, be fed from more than 10^6 B-lineage-committed progenitors and from stem cells. Very little is known of the forces that drive this early expansion of cells towards the B lineage, which should be antigen-independent, polyclonal and self-renewing, and might occur in fetal liver and bone marrow in contact with stromal cells.

In search of this large proliferative pool of progenitors and their growth requirement "in vivo" and "in vitro" we have developed reagents which detect early precursor B cells. A monoclonal antibody, called G-5-2, identifies precursor B cells more specifically than all other monoclonal antibodies available to date (Strasser, 1988). With the aid of this monoclonal antibody the growth properties of cell-sorter-enriched populations of pre B cells from fetal liver have been studied in response to single interleukin 1, or 2, or 3, or 4, or 5, or combinations of them (Karasuyama and Melchers, 1988). In parallel, we have begun to identify precursor B cell-specific genes which are found in cDNA libraries subtracted by mRNA from T cells (Sakaguchi, Berger and Melchers, 1986; Sakaguchi and Melchers, 1986; Kudo, Sakaguchi and Melchers, 1987; Kudo and Melchers, 1987; Kudo et al., 1987; Bauer, Kudo and Melchers, 1988). Three genes are described in some detail.

G-5-2, A MONOCLONAL ANTIBODY WITH A NOVEL PATTERN OF SPECIFICITY FOR CELLS OF THE B LINEAGE.

Hybridoma G-5-2 was raised in a fusion of the Ig-nonproducing hybridoma Sp2/0 with B cells activated in an alloreactive response by helper T cells of one parent transferred into an F_1 host, leading to graft-versus host disease and autoantibody production with lupus-like syndromes (Gleichmann et al., 1984; Rolink, Radaskiewicz and Melchers, 1987). The monoclonal antibody produced by one of the hybridomas was found to bind to a series of transformed pre B cell lines and to plasmacytomas, but not to mature, surface Ig-positive B cell lines, nor to cells of other lineages, such as T cells, macrophages, fibroblasts and progenitor cells (Table I). Binding studies to normal cells from fetal liver, bone marrow, spleen and lymph nodes in resting or antigen-stimulated states confirm this pattern of specificity. Consequently, it was possible to employ this monoclonal antibody for the enrichment by fluorescence-activated cell sorting of both, antigen-activated, Ig-secreting cells from spleen, and of surface Ig-negative pre B cells from fetal liver.

POSSIBLE DIFFERENCES IN THE DEVELOPMENT OF PRE B CELLS "IN VIVO" AND "IN VITRO".

Cells sorted from fetal liver for binding to the G-5-2 mAb were enriched for cells expressing mRNA for μH chain and, as a specific marker for pre B cells (see below), for λ_5, as detected by "in situ" hybridization of single cells with the appropriate radiolabelled probes (Berger, 1986) (Table II). These cells were also enriched for pre B cells which develop "in vitro" in the presence of rat thymus filler cells and the polyclonal activator lipopolysaccharide (LPS) (Melchers, 1977), in the same time as "in vivo", to clones of Ig-secreting, plaque forming cells, enumerated as frequencies of cells in a given population by limiting dilution analyses. Enrichment of G-5-2 positive cells lead to a similarily high enrichment of λ_5-expressing cells. If all G-5-2 positive, λ_5-expressing cells of fetal liver belong to the B lineage then it is surprising that at day 14 of gestation only one in 3000 of such cells developed into a clone of plaque forming cells, while at day 18 one in 10 did. This 300-fold difference in frequencies might suggest either that not all G-5-2 positive λ_5-expressing cells belong to the B lineage, a suspicion for which no other evidence is available at present. It might alternatively indicate that development between day 14 and 18 of gestation of G-5-2 positive, λ_5-expressing pre B cells with productive rearrangements of the Ig H and L chain loci leading to expression of Ig and, therefore in the end, to a clone of cells detectable in a plaque assay, is different "in vivo" from "in vitro". There might be selection "in vivo" of cells with productively rearranged Ig genes, which does not occur "in vitro". Alternatively pre B cells may not continue to rearrange their Ig gene loci "in vitro" as they do "in vivo".

GROWTH OF G-5-2 POSITIVE PRE B CELLS FROM FETAL LIVER "IN VITRO" IN DEPENDENCE OF DIFFERENT INTERLEUKINS.

G-5-2 positive cells from fetal liver at day 16 of gestation, enriched by fluorescence-activated cell sorting with the mAb, were kept in tissue culture in the presence of different interleukins (IL) in serum-substituted medium (Iscove and Melchers, 1978). Single recombinant IL's were obtained from cell lines which were transfected with a bovine papilloma virus-based vector containing single cDNA genes of either IL-2, IL-3, IL-4, IL-5, or IL-6. These cell lines secrete constitutively large quantities of single IL's into the supernatant tissue culture medium (Karasuyama and Melchers, 1988). Human IL-1, produced by a bacterial vector, was obtained from Dr. Lomedico, Research Laboratories, F. Hoffmann-LaRoche Ltd, Nutley, N.J., USA. Of all possible combinations of IL's only those containing IL-3 and IL-4 induced the continous logarithmic growth of a majority of G-5-2 positive fetal liver cells for at least 4 days of culture. IL-3 and 4 together were optimal; the presence of IL-5 began to be inhibitory for growth at day 3 to 4 of culture. When LPS was added to cells growing in IL-3 plus 4 IgM secreting cells developed at day 7 to 9 of culture. These initial experiments on the growth conditions of pre B cells support previous findings that have shown IL-3 and 4 to be active in pre B

Table 1. Binding of mAb G-5-2 on Transformed Cell Lines.

CELL		STATUS OF Ig REARRANGEMENT		STATUS OF Ig EXPRESSION		G-5-2 EXPRESSION
		H chains	L chains	H chains	L chains	
PROGENITOR	416-B	R	G	-	-	- -
	HAFTL-1	R	G	-	-	- -
PRE-B	40-E1	R	G	-	-	+++
	220-8	R	G	-	-	+++
	204-1-8	R	G	-	-	++
	230-238	R	G	-	-	-
	28C-9	R	G	-	-	++
	204-3-1	R	G	+	-	+
	18-81	R	R	+	-	+++
	70Z/3	R	R	+	(-)	+
	38C 13	R	R	+	+	+
	HAFTL-1 pre-B	R	R	+	+	++
MATURE B	WEHI 279	R	R	+	+	(+)
	WEHI 231	R	R	+	+	-
	L10 A62	R	R	+	+	-
	K46R	R	R	+	+	-
	A20/3	R	R	+	+	-
	BALENLM17	R	R	+	+	-
	2PK3	R	R	+	+	-
PLASMA CELL	J558/L	R	R	-	+	+++
	MPC11	R	R	+	+	+
	Sp2/0	D	D	-	-	-
	X63	R	R	+	+	++
T CELLS	EL4					-
	BW5147					-
	K62					-
	SPH					-
	BDF_1					-
MYELOID	P388D1					-
	WEHI 3					-
	HAFTL-1 myeloid					-
FIBRO-BLASTS	Ltk^-					-
	NIH3T3					-

G = Germ line
R = Rearranged
D = Deleted

Table 2. Frequencies of LPS-Reactive Precursors in λ_5-Positive, G-2-5-Positive Cells From Fetal Liver at Different Stages of Embryonic Development.

DAY OF GESTATION	% λ_5-POSITIVE CELLS		PRECURSORS OF LPS-REACTIVE CELLS	
	Of total	In G-T-2 enriched population	Of total	In G-T-2 enriched population
day 14	1	50–60	1 in 10^6	1 in 3000
day 16	3.3	70–80	1 in 10^4	1 in 250
day 18	5.7	>90	1 in 10^2	1 in 10

to B cell development (Palacios et al., 1984) and suggest that IL-3 plus 4 can stimulate pre B cells to become LPS- reactive B cells, probably in a time "in vitro" (2 to 3 days after day 16 of gestation) similar to the time of development "in vivo", a program which has been observed in previous "in vitro" experiments (Melchers, 1977).

B LINEAGE-RELATED GENES, WHICH ARE SELECTIVELY EXPRESSED AT THE PRE B CELL STAGE

For a search of genes which might be expressed at a given stage in the B lymphocyte development pathway and which might function to control this development we constructed a cDNA library from a pre B lymphoma cell. We subtracted sequences also present in a T cell hybridoma and probed the remaining two hundred cDNA clones with poly A^+ RNA from a panel of pre B, B, plasmacytoma, macrophage, fibroblast cell lines and with L cells for lineage-related, stage-specific expression. So far, we have identified three genes, called $V_{preB}1$, $V_{preB}2$ and λ_5, which are selectively expressed in pre B cell lines and normal pre B cells, but not in mature B cells, in plasmacytomas and Ig-secreting cells, nor in cells of other hemopoietic lineages and fibroblasts. Expression was estimated to be of medium to low abundance, with approximately fifty DNA copies per cell, detectable by "in situ" hybridization with specific radiolabeled probes.

Expression is first detected in cells, which begin to rearrange their Ig H chain genes, i.e. which rearrange D_H to J_H segments. The three genes continue to be expressed throughout pre B cell development in the $Ly1^+$ and $Ly1^-$ lineages. They are no longer detectable in normal B cells and in most Ig-positive B cell lines and remain not expressed as B cells mature to Ig-secreting plasma cells. Expression of λ_5 is, however, not down-regulated by the productive rearrangements of Ig H chain and L chain genes, nor by the deposition of Ig in the surface membrane, since two virus-tranformed pre B cell lines (NFS-5, 300-19) which continue to rearrange Ig gene loci and finally become surface Ig-positive, nevertheless, continue to express the pre B specific genes. These genes are, therefore, markers for pre B cells which are independent of the state of Ig-gene rearrangements (Sakaguchi, N.; Kudo, A.; Thalmann, P.; Davidson, W.; Pierce, J.H. and Melchers, F. manuscript submitted for publication).

THE STRUCTURES OF THE THREE PRE B RELATED GENES

The cDNA sequences of the three genes expressed in pre B- lymphocytes, and the intron-exon structures of their genomic forms have been determined (Sakaguchi and Melchers, 1986; Kudo, Sakaguchi and Melchers, 1987; Kudo and Melchers, 1987). The gene λ_5 is encoded by three exons, two of which show strong sequence homologies with λ L chains. In fact, the third exon is highly homologous to the constant region domain of λL chains, while the second exon shows strong homologies to J-sequences of λ L chain and to intron sequences 5' of the J λ -sequences. Homology to λ L chain gene segments is lost at the 5' end of the second exon of λ_5, so that the first exon of λ_5 and the intron in between the first and the second exon show no homologies to any known DNA sequences.

Approximately 4.2 kb upstream of the λ_5 gene is the $V_{preB}1$ gene. It consists of two exons. The first exon shows strong homology to sequences encoding the leader peptide of λ L chain, so do sequences of the intron between the first and the second exon to intron sequences between the leader and the variable region sequences of λL chain genes. The second exon, for most of its 5' part shows weak, but significant homologies to V region sequences of V_H, V_K and Vλ gene segments. At its 3' end, homologies to V-region sequences are lost. In fact, these 3' sequences of the second exon and the adjacent intron sequences 3' of the second exon have no detectable homology or similarity to any known DNA sequences.

The three genes, $V_{preB}1$, $V_{preB}2$ and λ_5, are located on chromosome 16 of the mouse, an unknown distance away from the gene segments encoding λL chains (Kudo et al, 1987).

The third gene, $V_{preB}2$, is almost identical to $V_{preB}1$. It has only few nucleotides different, some of which result in coding changes. Both $V_{preB}1$ and $V_{preB}2$ are expressed in pre B cells, as probing with specific oligonucleotides has shown. As $V_{preB}1$, and λ_5, $V_{preB}2$ is also located on mouse chromosome 16. The exact location relative to $V_{preB}1$ and λ_5, or to the λL chain genes is, however, not known.

In the human, V_{preB} is found within a cluster of V segments encoding the variable regions of human λL genes on chromosome 22. The human counterpart of V_{preB} has been cloned and sequenced (Bauer, Kudo and Melchers, 1988). A remarkable conservation of sequences is observed in nucleotide positions corresponding to frameworks 2 and 3 of V-gene segments. Thus, a stretch of 59 nucleotides in framework 2 is identical, and only 10 nucleotide exchanges in a stretch of 97 nucleotides of framework 3 are found between the mouse and the human sequence. Similar sequence homologies are likely to exist for other mammalian species, since Southern blots of DNA from calf, rabbit, rat, guinea pig and hamster show bands crosshybridizing with the mouse V_{preB} probe under high stringency. Furthermore, a remarkable conservation of the gene structure of and around V_{preB} is detected by the fact, that very little restriction length polymorphism is detectable within a species. None of these genes are rearranged during B cell development.

Proteins encoded by the three genes have so far not been detected, although λ_5 and $V_{preB}1$ have been expressed both in bacterial and animals cells by tranfection with appropriate expression vectors containing the corresponding cDNA genes. We can, therefore, only speculate what the function of V_{preB} and λ_5 might be.

It appears possible that V_{preB} may associate by noncovalent interactions with a λ_5 protein, forming, at the site of the third complementarity determining region of a comparable V-region of Ig molecules, a large protrusion consisting of the amino terminal portion of λ_5 encoded by the 5' portion of the λ_5 gene, and by the carboxy terminal portion of V_{preB}, encoded by the 3' portion of the gene, both of which show no sequence homology to any known gene. This might represent a constant binding site expressed in all pre B cells.

λ_5 with its c-region-like domain, including the penultimate cysteine at the carboxy terminal end, could well associate convalently with a μ H-chain in pre B cells, as soon as H chains (VDJ or DJ protein) are expressed. The ternary complex of $V_{preB}1$, λ_5 and μH chain could well appear on the surface of pre B cells (Melchers, Andersson and Phillips, 1977) where it may perform binding functions via the protrusion at the boundary of V_{preV} and λ_5 which is constant for all pre B cells, and which might control pre B development and function in interactions with stromal cells.

ACKNOWLEDGEMENTS

We thank Ms. Heidi Brächtold, Annick Peter, Denise Richterich Guex and Mr. Wyn Davies for able technical assistance. The Basel Institute for Immunology was founded and is supported by F. Hoffmann-LaRoche & Co, Ltd.

REFERENCES

Berger, C.N. (1986) EMBO J. 5, 85-93.
Bauer, S.R., Kudo, A. and Melchers, F. (1988) EMBO J. 7, 111-116.
Gleichmann, E.; Pals, S.T.; Rolink, T.; Radaskiewicz, T. and Gleichmann, H. (1984) Immunology Today 5, 324-327.
Iscove, N.N. and Melchers, F. (1978) J. Expo. Med. 147, 923-929.
Karasuyama, H. and Melchers, F. (1988) Eur. J. Immunol. 18, 97-104.
Kudo, A. and Melchers, F. (1987) EMBO J. 6, 103-107.

Kudo, A.; Pravtcheva, D.; Sakaguchi, N.; Ruddle, F. and Melchers, F. (1987) Genomics 1, 277-279.
Kudo, A., Sakaguchi, N. and Melchers, F. (1987) EMBO J. 6, 103-107.
Melchers, F (1977) Eur. J. Immunol. 7, 476-487.
Melchers, F.; Andersson, J. and Phillips, R.A. (1977) Cold Spring Harbor, Symp. Quant. Biol. 41, 147-158.
Osmond, D.G. (1986) Immunol. Rev. 93, 105-124.
Palacios, R.; Hanson, G.; Steinmetz, M. and McKearn, J.P. (1984) Nature 309, 126-131.
Rolink, A.G.; Radaskiewicz, T. and Melchers, F. (1987) J. Expo. Med. 165, 1675-1687.
Sakaguchi, N.; Berger, C.N. and Melchers, F. (1986) EMBO J. 5, 2139-2147.
Sakaguchi, N. and Melchers, F. (1986) Nature 324, 579-582.
Strasser, A. (1988) Ph.D. Thesis, University of Basel, Switzerland.

G-PROTEIN REGULATION OF POLYPHOSPHOINOSITIDE BREAKDOWN IN B CELLS

G.G.B. Klaus, M.M. Harnett and K.P. Rigley

National Institute for Medical Research
Mill Hill, London NW7 1AA, UK

INTRODUCTION

It is now well-established that antigen receptors on both T and B lymphocytes belong to the large group of widely distributed Ca^{2+}-mobilizing receptors. In other words, crosslinking of these receptors by anti-receptor antibodies, or antigens, activates a polyphosphoinositide-specific phosphodiesterase (PPI-PDE), whose primary substrate is phosphatidyl-inositol 4,5 bisphosphate (PIP_2). This is broken down to inositol 1,4,5-trisphosphate (IP_3) and 1,2 diacylglycerol. IP_3 causes the release of Ca^{2+} from intracellular stores, and diacylglycerol is an essential co-factor for the Ca^{2+} and phospholipid dependent protein kinase C (PKC). In B cells, as in many other cell types, both arms of this branched signalling pathway are required to generate an optimal biological response, in this case activation of resting cells into the cell cycle: this has been demonstrated by the synergistic effects of Ca^{2+} ionophores and PKC-activating phorbol esters in inducing DNA synthesis in both human and murine B cells. Recent reviews on signalling by surface immunoglobulin (sIg) receptors on B cells can be found in refs. 1 and 2.

Signal transduction by receptors which utilize cAMP as a second messenger system is known to be controlled by stimulatory (G_s) and inhibitory (G_i) guanine nucleotide regulatory proteins, which couple the receptors to the catalytic effector, namely adenylate cyclase (reviewed in 3). It has recently become increasingly evident that Ca^{2+}-mobilizing receptors are also coupled to the PPI-PDE via one or more types of G-protein, generically known as G_p (reviewed in 4). In line with this, we will present evidence here that both sIgM and sIgD receptors on mouse B cells are coupled to the PPI-PDE via an as yet unidentified G-protein. These results will be published in full elsewhere[5].

Murine B cells can be induced to synthesize DNA by high concentrations of $F(ab')_2$ fragments of rabbit anti-Ig antibodies, but not by their intact (IgG) counterparts. This is because the intact antibodies co-crosslink sIg and Fc gamma receptors (FcR) on B lymphocytes, and this generates an inhibitory signal that aborts B cell activation[6,7] and antigen receptor-stimulated PIP_2 hydrolysis[8].
The nature of the inhibitory signal generated via the FcR is therefore of considerable interest, since this system is believed to provide a model for the regulation of B cell activation by antigen-IgG antibody complexes, or by anti-idiotypic antibodies. We

present evidence that co-crosslinking sIg and FcR uncouples sIg receptors from the putative G-protein involved in activation of the PPI-PDE (K.P. Rigley and G.G.B. Klaus, in preparation).

G-PROTEIN COUPLING OF sIg RECEPTORS TO THE PPI-PDE

A classical way of demonstrating G-protein involvement in signalling is to mimic receptor activation by introducing non-hydrolyzable GTP analogues, such as GTPγS, into permeabilized cells. Permeabilization effectively uncouples G-protein linked receptors, because the cells lose endogenous GTP, and the system can be reconstituted by such GTP analogues, which irreversibly activate all G-proteins in the cell. Thus, a series of experiments were undertaken in which [^{3}H]-inositol-labelled, purified mouse B cells were permeabilized with streptolysin 0, and then stimulated at various Ca^{2+} concentrations with GTPγS, in the presence or absence of anti-Ig antibodies. GTPγS alone induced dose-dependent release of [^{3}H]-inositol phosphates (including IP_3), thereby demonstrating the presence of G_p in B cells. Fig. 1 shows the results of a typical coupling experiment with polyclonal $F(ab')_2$ anti-Fab antibodies, over a range of Ca^{2+} concentrations from 100 nM to 10 uM. It is evident that in permeabilized B cells the PPI-PDE is virtually inactive at physiological Ca^{2+} concentrations, and is only weakly stimulated by anti-Ig alone. GTPγS induced release of inositol phosphates, which increased with increasing Ca^{2+} concentration, and this response was markedly augmented by co-stimulation with anti-Ig. These results, therefore formally demonstrate the involvement of G_p in polyphosphoinositide hydrolysis provoked by sIg crosslinking.

Do IgM and IgD Receptors Use the Same G-Protein?

To investigate whether both sIgM and sIgD receptors are G_p-linked, similar experiments were performed with monoclonal anti-u or anti-δ antibodies, with comparable results (not shown). We therefore wished to study if both types of receptor utilize the same or different G-proteins. Two approaches have thus far been employed. The first was to use microbial toxins, which have been utilized with success in defining the properties of G_s (ADP-ribosylated by cholera toxin) and G_i (modified by pertussis toxin). It is known that the activity of G_p can be modified by pertussis toxin in some cell types, but not in others, thus suggesting that there are multiple forms of G_p (reviewed in 4). Pretreatment of B cells with 100 ng/ml pertussis toxin had no effects on PIP_2 breakdown induced by either anti-u or anti-δ antibodies, thereby demonstrating that G_p in B cells is not G_i-like. Treatment of B cells with cholera toxin caused some 30% inhibition of inositol phosphate release provoked by anti-Fab, anti-u or anti-δ antibodies. The significance of this finding is difficult to interpret, but we think it unlikely that G_p in B cells is G_s-like. Rather, these effects of cholera toxin probably reflect elevation of cAMP levels resulting from activation of G_s, since similar partial inhibition can be induced by cAMP analogues.

We have recently shown[9] that very low doses of cholera toxin (ca. 10^{-14}M) inhibit DNA synthesis (but not increases in Ia antigen levels) in murine B cells cultured with by $F(ab')_2$ anti-Ig: this effect is highly selective, in that lipopolysaccharide-stimulated B cell proliferation is only suppressed by concentrations of toxin several orders of magnitude higher. Paradoxically, levels of toxin which inhibit anti-Ig responses enhance DNA synthesis induced by phorbol esters plus Ca^{2+} ionophore. The mechanisms involved are unclear, but these phenomena are unlikely to simply reflect elevation of cAMP levels by cholera toxin, since other cAMP agonists do not show anywhere near the same degree of selectivity. We favor the idea that the toxin, besides its well-known effects on G_s, also modifies an additional G-protein involved further downstream in the activation cascade induced by anti-Ig.

The second approach we have used to attempt to identify multiple forms of G_p in B cells is to study the influence of PKC-activating phorbol esters, such as phorbol myristic acetate (PMA) on receptor signalling. These agents are known to inhibit receptor-stimulated PIP_2 hydrolysis in various cells, including B cells[10, 11],

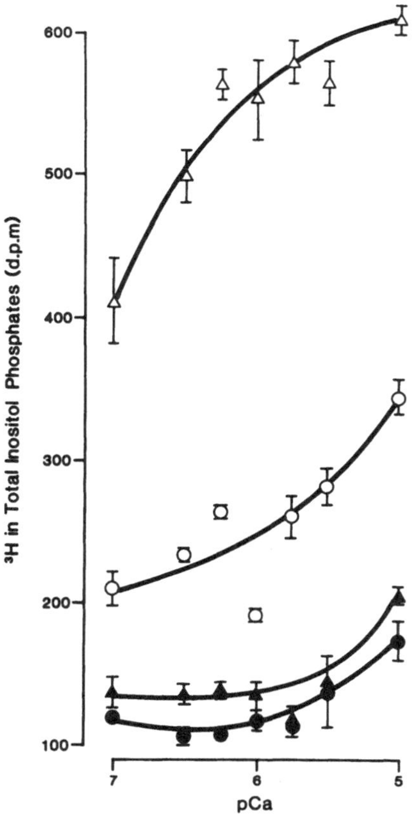

Fig. 1. Coupling of sIg receptors to the PPI-PDE via G_p. Purified B cells were labelled with $[^3H]$-inositol, permeabilized with streptolysin 0, transferred to Ca^{2+} buffers as indicated (pCa 7 = 100 nM) and were then stimulated with Ca^{2+} alone (●), 100 uM GTP S (O), 50 ug/ml $F(ab')_2$ anti-Fab antibodies (▲), or GTPγS + anti-Ig (Δ). Release of total inositol phosphates was determined after 10 min. See ref. 5.

and this has been reported to be due to uncoupling of receptors from G_p in some systems[12]. Dose-response titrations of PMA in intact B cells showed that this agent inhibits both basal inositol phosphate release, and responses stimulated by anti-u or anti-δ antibodies equally well (data not shown). The effects of PMA on responses to GTPγS in the presence or absence of isotype-specific antibodies in permeabilized B cells are summarized in Table 1. These experiments showed that 160 nM PMA inhibits basal $[^3H]$-inositol phosphate release, and responses provoked by any of the stimuli, alone or in combination, equally well, i.e., by about 65-70%.

The results summarized above suggest (but by no means prove) that sIgM and sIgD receptors share a common species of (and perhaps the same) G-protein, since the signalling provoked by anti-u or anti-δ antibodies was not differentially affected by pertussis or cholera toxins, or by PMA. Thus again, experiments with isotype-specific antibodies have failed to provide any more clues to one of the fundamental mysteries of B cell biology, namely, why most of these cell express at least two classes of sIg. The effects of PMA are difficult to interpret: clearly the agent has profound inhibitory

Table 1. Effects of PMA on inositol phospholipid degradation in permeabilized B cells.

Stimuli: [a]	[^{3}H]-inositol phosphate release (% of total radioactivity): [b] Controls:	PMA:
pCa7	1.05 ± 0.04	0.35 ± 0.02 (67)
GTPγS	1.41 ± 0.03	0.41 ± 0.02 (71)
Anti-u	1.40 ± 0.02	0.47 ± 0.1 (68)
Anti-δ	1.63 ± 0.06	0.50 ± 0.03 (70)
GTPγS + anti-u	1.94 ± 0.1	0.66 ± 0.02 (66)
GTPγS + anti-δ	2.2 ± 0.1	0.72 ± 0.07 (67)

a) [^{3}H]-inositol-labelled B cells were incubated (10 min., 37°C) with medium or 160 nM PMA, and then permeabilized for 5 min. with streptolysin 0, when the indicated additions were made (in buffer at pCa 7): GTPγS (10 uM), with or without 50 ug/ml monoclonal anti-u or anti-δ antibodies.

b) Total [^{3}H]-inositol phosphates were determined after a further 10 min. incubation. Figures in brackets give the percentage inhibition caused by PMA. Results are means ± SEM (n = 3) from a representative experiment.

effects on both basal and receptor-stimulated inositol phospholipid breakdown in B cells. However, unlike recent findings with angiotensin receptors on mesangial cells[12], in B cells PMA obviously does not uncouple sIg receptors from G_p. Instead, the inhibition of inositol phospholipid breakdown in these cells caused by phorbol esters may be a consequence of PKC activation inhibiting the PPI-PDE, or one or more of the PI kinases, thereby resulting in a general suppression of the PI cycle.

UNCOUPLING OF sIg RECEPTORS FROM G_p BY ENGAGING Fc RECEPTORS

Intact (IgG) rabbit anti-Ig antibodies cause a short-lived burst of IP_3 release in B cells, which is abrogated after about 1 minute[8]. Furthermore, intact anti-Ig antibodies inhibit both inositol phospholipid breakdown and DNA synthesis induced by the $F(ab')_2$ fragments[6-8]. Various mechanisms can be envisaged whereby co-crosslinking of sIg and FcR by such antibodies could shut down PIP_2 hybrolysis, and two of these possibilities are readily testable in permeabilized B cells. If engaging FcR has a direct inhibitory effect on the PPI-PDE, then intact anti-Ig should depress inositol phosphate release provoked by GTPγS either alone, or in combination with $F(ab')_2$ anti-Ig. On the other hand, if the FcR acts by uncoupling sIg from G_p, then only <u>coupled</u> responses to $F(ab')_2$ anti-Fab Ig plus GTPγS should be suppressed, but not the response to the GTP analogue on its own.

The results of a typical experiment designed to test these two hypotheses are shown in Fig. 2. [^{3}H]-inositol-labelled, permeabilized B cells were equilibrated to 100 nM Ca^{2+} (pCa 7) and were stimulated with $F(ab')_2$ anti-Fab antibodies, in the presence, or absence, or IgG anti-Ig and increasing concentrations of GTPγS. The intact antibodies induced weak co-stimulation with GTPγS, presumably reflecting continuing low level PIP_2 breakdown seen previously in intact cells[8]. Mixing $F(ab')_2$ anti-Ig with intact antibodies (at a molar ratio of 1.0 : 0.5) inhibited the coupled response to $F(ab')_2$ anti-Ig, to the residual level given by the intact antibodies. Significantly, the suppression never exceeded the level of response given by GTPγS alone. This phenomenon was seen over a range of Ca^{2+} concentrations, and with a wide range of intact antibody concentrations.

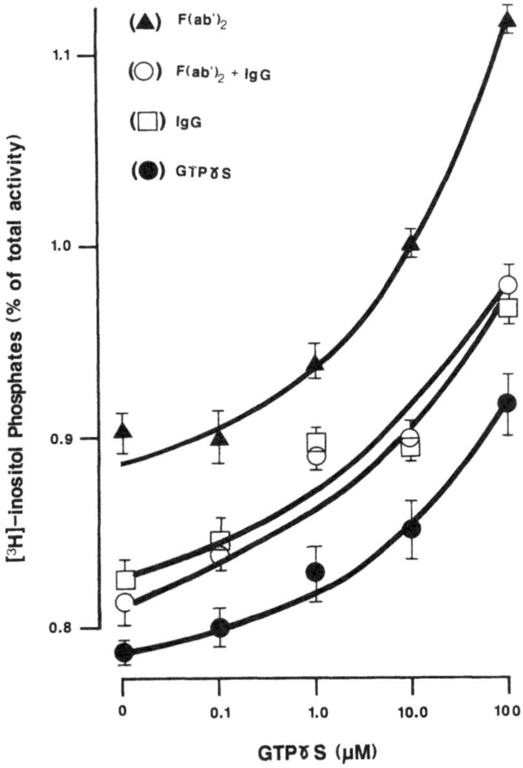

Fig. 2. Uncoupling of sIg from G_p by engaging FcR. [^{3}H]-inositol-labelled permeabilized B cells at pCa 7 were stimulated with 50 ug/ml $F(ab')_2$ anti-Fab, or 37.5 ug/ml IgG anti-Fab, alone or in combination, in the presence of 0-100 uM GTPγS. Release of total inositol phosphates was determined after 10 min. Results are means ± SEM (n = 3) from a representative experiment. (K.P. Rigley and G.G.B. Klaus, in prep.).

We interpret these results as follows. Co-crosslinking of sIg and FcR by intact anti-Ig antibodies leads to uncoupling of sIg receptors from G_p, and has no detectable effects on the coupling of G_p to the PPI-PDE, or on the PPI-PDE itself. The mechanisms involved remain to be elucidated. Various possibilities can be envisaged, e.g., activation of a protein kinase by ligation of the FcR, and consequent phosphorylation of G_p, or simple physical uncoupling of sIg from G_p by the intact antibodies. The latter is a particularly attractive hypothesis, given the evidence for some sort of physical association between FcR and sIg receptors within the plane of the B cell membrane[13].

CONCLUSIONS

The data summarized here demonstrate that both sIgM and sIgD receptors on B cells are coupled to their second messenger generating system via a form of G_p. The nature of the protein still remains to be established: it could be a classical heterotrimeric type of G-protein (like G_s and G_i), or it could be of the p21 ras type, which has been proposed to couple bombesin receptors to the PPI-PDE in fibroblasts[14]. It is also still uncertain if different sIg isotypes on B cells utilize the same or separate G-proteins. However, it is clear that the G_p(s) in B cells are not substrates for pertussis toxin, and neither are they directly affected by PKC-activating phorbol esters. In addition, we have demonstrated that engaging FcR and sIg together leads to uncoupling of sIg receptors from G_p: these findings afford a mechanistic explanation for the inhibitory effects of intact anti-Ig, both on signalling via sIg receptors and on B cell activation by $F(ab')_2$ anti-Ig. By extrapolation, these results should also be relevant to the FcR-mediated inhibitory effects of antigen-antibody complexes and anti-idiotypic antibodies on B cell activation by specific antigen (reviewed in 15).

REFERENCES

1. J. C. Cambier, L. B. Justement, M.K. Newell, Z. Z. Chen, L. K. Harris, V. Sandoval, M. J. Klemsz and J. T. Ransom, Immunol. Rev. 95: 37 (1987).
2. G. G. B. Klaus, M. K. Bijsterbosch, A. O'Garra, M. M. Harnett and K. P. Rigley, Immunol. Rev. 99: 19 (1987).
3. A. G. Gilman, Cell 36: 577 (1984).
4. S. Cockcroft, Trends Biochem. Sci. 12: 75 (1987).
5. M. M. Harnett and G. G. B. Klaus, J. Immunol. 140: 3135 (1988).
6. N. E. Phillips and D. C. Parker, J. Immunol. 132: 627 (1984).
7. G. G. B. Klaus, C. M. Hawrylowicz, M. Holman and K. D. Keeler, Immunology 53: 693 (1984).
8. M. K. Bijsterbosch and G. G. B. Klaus, J. Exp. Med. 162: 1825 (1985).
9. G. G. B. Klaus, K. Vondy and M. Holman, Eur. J. Immunol. 17: 1787 (1987).
10. J. Mizuguchi, M. A. Beavan, J. H. Li and W. E. Paul, Proc. Nat. Acad. Sci. USA 83: 4474 (1986).
11. M. K. Bijsterbosch and G. G. B. Klaus, Eur. J. Immunol. 17: 113 (1987).
12. J. Pfeilschifter and C. Bauer, Biochem. J. 248: 209 (1987).
13. A. K. Abbas and E. R. Unanue, J. Immunol. 115: 1665 (1975).
14. M. J. Wakelam, S. A. Davies and M. D. Houslay, Nature 323: 173 (1986).
15. N. R. St.C. Sinclair and A. Panaskoltsis, Immunol. Today 8: 76 (1987).

SIGNAL TRANSDUCTION VIA THE B CELL ANTIGEN RECEPTOR: INVOLVEMENT OF A G PROTEIN AND REGULATION OF SIGNALING

Anthony L. DeFranco and Michael R. Gold

Departments of Microbiology and Immunology and
Biochemistry and Biophysics,
University of California, San Francisco, San Francisco, CA 94143-0552

INTRODUCTION

The antigen receptor on B lymphocytes plays critical roles in B cell development and B cell activation. Antigen or anti-immunoglobulin stimulation of membrane IgM (mIgM) on immature B cells, such as those found in neonatal mice, results in the functional inactivation of the B cell[1]. This response, referred to as "clonal anergy" by Nossal and colleagues, would be expected to inactivate B cells with mIgM specific for autoantigens in the environment of the developing B cell, and hence may play a role in the generation of B cell tolerance. Stimulation of the antigen receptor on a mature B cell, on the other hand, contributes to the activation of that cell to proliferate and differentiate into antibody secreting cells[2,3]. In the case of the immature B cell, the antigen receptor must be acting as a signal transducing receptor, since this response can be seen at the single cell level[4]. In the case of B cell activation, mIg appears to play a dual role: it can serve as a very efficient means of taking up antigen for presentation to helper T cells[5-7]. Additionally, mIg can act as a signal transducing receptor, as revealed by the striking effects of anti-immunoglobulin antibodies on resting mature B cells[8].

In its action as a signal transducing receptor, membrane immunoglobulin acts by triggering the breakdown of a plasma membrane phospholipid, phosphatidylinositol 4,5-bisphosphate (PIP_2)[9]. This breakdown is accomplished by a phospholipase C specific for phosphatidylinositol, especially the phosphorylated forms such as PIP_2. The released second messengers are diacylglycerol (DG), which activates protein kinase C, and inositol(1,4,5) trisphosphate ($InsP_3$), which causes the release of calcium from internal stores[10]. It had been shown by the pioneering work of Braun et al. and Pozzan et al.[11,12] that anti-Ig causes a rise in cytoplasmic calcium concentration. This increase results from PIP_2 breakdown, rather than vice versa, since, when extracellular calcium is removed, the calcium increase is decreased in magnitude and duration, yet the PIP_2 breakdown response is largely unaffected[13].

Cytoplasmic free calcium and diacylglycerol are thought to be the important second messengers generated by PIP_2 hydrolysis. For example, elevation of Ca^{2+} with calcium ionophores and activation of protein kinase C with phorbol esters mimics the action of anti-IgM on mature B cells, at least to some extent[14-17]. We have examined this issue in WEHI-231 B lymphoma cells, where anti-Ig also induces PIP_2 breakdown, as well as causing growth arrest[13,18,19]. Here phorbol dibutyrate and ionomycin can induce a growth arrest which is similar to that induced by anti-IgM, although it is slower. Furthermore, anti-IgM induces a decrease in cell size in addition to growth arrest, whereas the mimicking reagents do not. Thus, in WEHI-231 cells calcium and diacylglycerol appear to be responsible for mediating some of the effects of mIgM signaling but not others (D.M. Page and A.L. DeFranco, Role of phosphoinositide-derived second messengers in mediating anti-IgM-induced growth arrest of WEHI-231 B lymphoma cells. J. Immunol. 140:3717 (1988)). It is possible that one of the inositol phosphate compounds plays a second messenger role in addition to causing the elevation of calcium. An attractive candidate in this regard is inositol(1,3,4,5) tetrakisphosphate ($InsP_4$). In several cell types, including WEHI-231[13], $InsP_3$ is phosphorylated to yield $InsP_4$. Furthermore, this compound has been shown to have biological effects on sea urchin oocyte activation[20] and on regulation of K^+ channels[21]. In any case, second messengers derived from phosphoinositide hydrolysis clearly play important roles in mediating the biological effects of mIgM signaling.

Given the central role of antigen receptor signaling in B cell activation and development, it seems likely that these reactions will be modulated by some of the many other signals impinging on the B cell. One clearcut example of this has already been described, the inhibition of mIg-induced phosphoinositide breakdown by simultaneous engagement of mIgM and the Fc receptor for IgG[22]. In order to be able to identify and understand such regulation in more detail, we have studied the mechanism by which mIgM activates the phosphoinositide-specific phospholipase C. We have demonstrated that an intermediary component exists, and that it has properties in common with the G protein family of receptor-effector coupling components seen in the adenylate cyclase and rhodopsin systems[23,24]. Furthermore, we have discovered a feedback inhibition of phosphoinositide breakdown. This inhibition was found to be mediated by protein kinase C. Here we describe recent experiments to determine the locus at which it acts in the signal transduction pathway.

RESULTS AND DISCUSSION

Involvement of a G Protein in Signaling by mIgM

We wanted to understand how crosslinking mIgM leads to activation of phospholipase C and hydrolysis of PIP_2. One clue came from biochemical studies of other transmembrane signaling reactions in mammalian cells. In several well characterized signaling systems, receptors are coupled to effector enzymes or ion channels by a family of GTP-binding proteins termed G proteins. The list of effectors which are activated by G proteins now includes adenylate cyclase, rhodopsin-stimulated cGMP phosphodiesterases in the visual system, K^+channels, and perhaps phospholipase A_2 [23,24]. We therefore examined whether a G protein was involved in signaling by mIgM.

The G proteins characterized thus far share a number of unique biochemical properties. Interaction of a G protein with a ligand-bound receptor causes the G protein to release GDP and to bind GTP. Binding GTP converts the G protein to an activated form that can regulate the activity of the corresponding effector. The G protein possesses an intrinsic GTPase activity that cleaves the GTP to GDP, returning the G protein to the inactive GDP-bound state. The GTPase activity is relatively slow, and this allows a single activated G protein to stimulate multiple reactions by the effector. This property allows G proteins to amplify receptor-stimulated reactions and may be the basis for the common use of G proteins in signal transduction systems. The biochemical properties of G proteins provide the following testable criteria for the involvement of a G protein in a reaction:

(1) The reaction requires GTP or GTP analogues
(2) The reaction is specific for GTP or GTP analogues
(3) The reaction is inhibited by GDP or GDP analogues.

To test these criteria, it was necessary to introduce guanine nucleotides into B cells. Since guanine nucleotides do not diffuse across the plasma membrane of cells, a low concentration (20 μg/ml) of the detergent saponin was used to permeabilize WEHI-231 B lymphoma cells. These permeabilized cells were found to take up trypan blue but remain intact for at least 1 hour at 37°C. The permeabilized cells were suspended in a

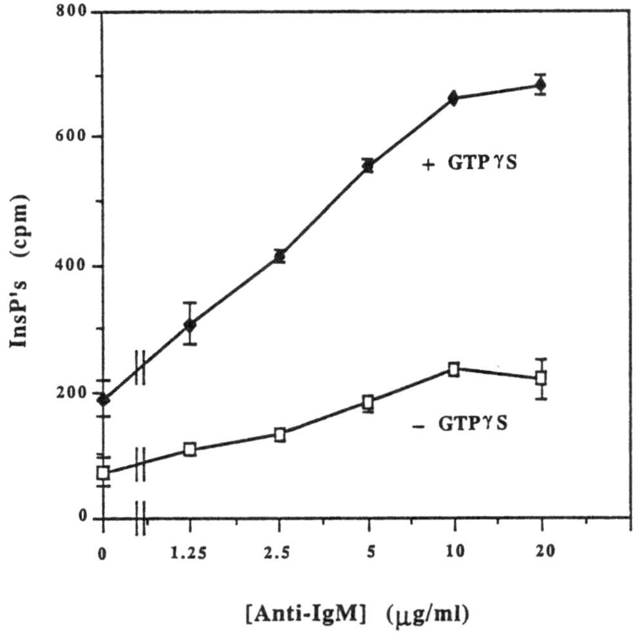

Figure 1. GTPγS increases signaling by mIgM in permeabilized WEHI-231 cells. Permeabilized WEHI-231 cells were incubated for 10 minutes with the indicated concentrations of a monoclonal anti-IgM antibody (Bet 1) in the presence or absence of 100 μM GTPγS. The production of total inositol phosphates was determined. The time zero value (inositol phosphate content of the permeabilized cells at the beginning of the reaction) subtracted from each experimental value was 432 cpm. Each data point is the average and range of duplicate samples. Reprinted from Gold et al.[25] by permission of the Journal of Immunology.

cytoplasm-like buffer (20 mM NaHepes, pH 7.2, 116 mM KCl, 4 mM NaCl, 5 mM $NaHCO_3$, 1 mM NaH_2PO_4, 2 mM MgC_{12}, 1 mM EGTA, 0.7 mM $CaCl_2$, 10 mM LiCl, 1 mM DTT, 2 mM MgATP) with a physiological concentration of free calcium (approx. 500 nM). Anti-IgM antibodies and various nucleotides were added and the reactions were allowed to proceed for 10 minutes. The inositol phosphates were then separated by ion exchange chromatography using Dowex AG-1-X8 columns[25]. This system allowed us to diffuse various nucleotides into the cells and examine their effects on phosphoinositide signaling by mIgM.

Figure 1 shows that addition of a non-hydrolyzable GTP analogue to the permeabilized WEHI-231 cells potentiated signaling by mIgM. In the absence of added guanine nucleotides, anti-IgM antibodies typically caused a 2-3 fold increase in the production of inositol phosphates. However, addition of GTPγS, a stable analogue of GTP, greatly increased the ability of anti-IgM to cause inositol phosphate production. GTPγS caused a small increase in inositol phosphate production by itself, but the effect of adding anti-IgM and GTPγS together was much more than additive. Only non-hydrolyzable analogues of GTP potentiated signaling by mIgM[25]. GDP and GDP analogues did not increase signaling by mIgM. In addition, the reaction was specific for guanine nucleotides, since ATPγS was also without effect.

The ability of stable GTP analogues to potentiate signaling by mIgM is consistent with the involvement of a G protein in this reaction. There were two observations, however, that were difficult to explain at first. One was that while GTPγS stimulated

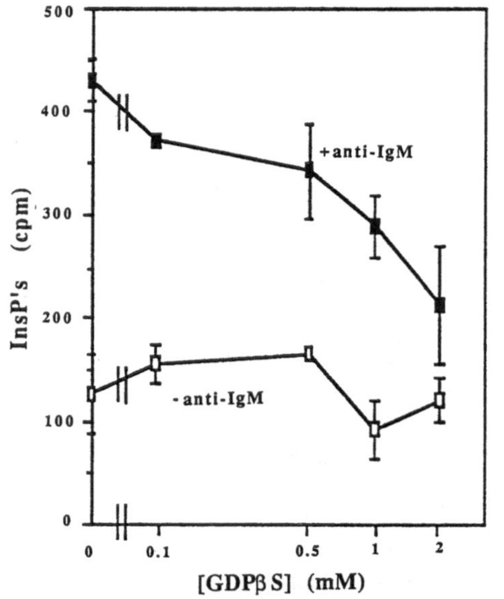

Figure 2. GDPßS inhibits signaling by mIgM. Permeabilized WEHI-231 cells were incubated for 10 minutes with or without 10 μg/ml of a monoclonal anti-IgM antibody (Bet 1) in the presence of the indicated concentrations of GDPßS. In the absence of GDPßS, the production of inositol phosphates in response to 10 μg/ml anti-IgM plus 100 μM GTPγS was 797 ± 15 cpm. The time zero value subtracted from each experimental point in this experiment was 722 cpm. Each point is the average and range of duplicate samples. Reprinted from Gold et al.[25] with the permission of the Journal of Immunology.

signaling by mIgM, GTP had no effect[25]. The second was that crosslinking mIgM did cause a modest increase in inositol phosphate production in the absence of any added guanine nucleotides (Figure 1). Both of these observations could be explained by proposing that the permeabilized cell system already contained significant amounts of GTP. These in vitro reactions employed a high concentration of ATP to maintain the phosphorylated state of PIP_2. The permeabilized cells may have been able to use the ATP to generate GTP. If the stimulation of inositol phosphate production by anti-IgM in the absence of added guanine nucleotides did involve a G protein utilizing endogenous GTP, then it should have been possible to inhibit this G protein by addition of GDPßS, a GDP analogue that cannot be converted to GTP. GDPßS inhibits reactions dependent on G proteins by competing with GTP for the nucleotide binding site of these proteins. Figure 2 shows that adding increasing concentrations of GDPßS did inhibit signaling by mIgM. This argues that the response to anti-IgM is G protein dependent and that there is endogenous GTP present to support the reaction.

Thus signaling by mIgM in this permeabilized cell system meets the criteria for a G protein-dependent reaction: It was stimulated by GTP analogues, was inhibited by GDP analogues, depended on GTP, and was specific for GTP and GTP analogues. Our results argue that crosslinking mIgM caused nucleotide exchange on a guanine nucleotide binding protein. In the absence of any added guanine nucleotides, crosslinking mIgM appeared to cause the release of GDP and the binding of endogenous GTP. In the presence of an excess of GDPßS, the GDPßS outcompeted the endogenous GTP for the nucleotide binding site and converted all the G proteins to an inactive state. Under these conditions signaling by mIgM was inhibited. When GTPγS was added to the reactions, crosslinking mIgM caused the binding of this nucleotide to the G protein. Since GTPγS cannot be hydrolyzed to GDP, the G protein stayed active for a much longer time than when GTP was bound, resulting in greater stimulation of phospholipase C.

Aluminum fluoride, a compound that activates the known G proteins, also stimulated production of inositol phosphates in permeabilized WEHI-231 cells (Table I) and in intact cells (data not shown). This result supports our hypothesis that phospholipase C activation in WEHI-231 cells is a G protein-dependent process.

The permeabilized cell system maintained a number of properties of the intact system. As seen in intact cells, inositol phosphate production was stimulated only by anti-IgM antibodies and not by anti-transferrin receptor antibodies or by anti-H-2 antibodies[25]. In addition, crosslinking mIgM on the permeabilized cells generated all four inositol phosphates (InsP, $InsP_2$, $InsP_3$, $InsP_4$) in relative amounts similar to those generated in intact cells (Table I).

The permeabilized cell system has also allowed us to examine the calcium requirement for phospholipase C activation by mIgM. Membrane Ig-mediated PIP_2 hydrolysis in permeabilized WEHI-231 cells required low levels of calcium. If the free calcium was reduced to less than 1 nM using EGTA, anti-IgM-stimulated PIP_2 breakdown was completely abolished[25]. Substantial anti-IgM-stimulated signaling was observed when calcium was maintained at 120 nM, the level found in unstimulated WEHI-231 cells. Slightly greater production of inositol phosphates was seen when the free calcium was adjusted to 500 nM, the level found in WEHI-231 cells after crosslinking mIgM. Thus the rapid, transient increase in cytosolic free calcium caused by crosslinking mIgM may potentiate receptor-stimulated PIP_2 breakdown somewhat. These results also show that phosphoinositide hydrolysis can occur prior to calcium elevation (i.e. at resting calcium levels, approx. 120 nM), consistent with evidence that PIP_2 breakdown precedes, and causes, the elevation of cytoplasmic calcium. Finally, very high, non-physiologic levels of calcium (> 100 μM) activated phospholipase C in the absence of crosslinking mIgM[25]. This is thought to be a direct effect on the phospholipase. As this mode of activation bypasses the G protein, it is a useful tool for determining the site of regulation of the phosphoinositide signaling pathway.

Table 1. Inositol Phosphate Production by Permeabilized WEHI-231 Cells.

	^{3}H-inositol phosphates				
Stimulus	InsP	$InsP_2$	$InsP_3$	$InsP_4$	Total InsP's
None	125 ± 19	75 ± 1	89 ± 9	34 ± 8	323 ± 19
NaF, 20 mM	252 ± 8	249 ± 25	288 ± 18	73 ± 3	861 ± 3
NaF, 10 mM	255 ± 15	169 ± 15	316 ± 3	49 ± 9	788 ± 4
NaF, 3 mM	146 ± 12	95 ± 3	120 ± 12	52 ± 7	413 ± 10
Anti-IgM, 10 μg/ml + GTPγS, 100 μM	376 ± 27	556 ± 70	895 ± 59	172 ± 12	2000 ± 29

[a] Permeabilized, ^{3}H-inositol-labelled WEHI-231 cells were incubated for 10 minutes with the indicated stimuli. Each point is the average and range of duplicate samples. For each sample the values for the four inositol phosphates were added together to determine the total inositol phosphates and the average and range for the totals is shown for the duplicate samples. All samples receiving NaF also included 10 M AlC_{13}. The inositol phosphate content of the cells at the beginning of the reaction was determined and these values were subtracted from the all the experimental values. In this experiment the "time zero" values were 316 cpm for InsP, 360 cpm for $InsP_2$, 397 cpm for $InsP_3$, 255 cpm for $InsP_4$ and 1328 cpm for the total InsP's.

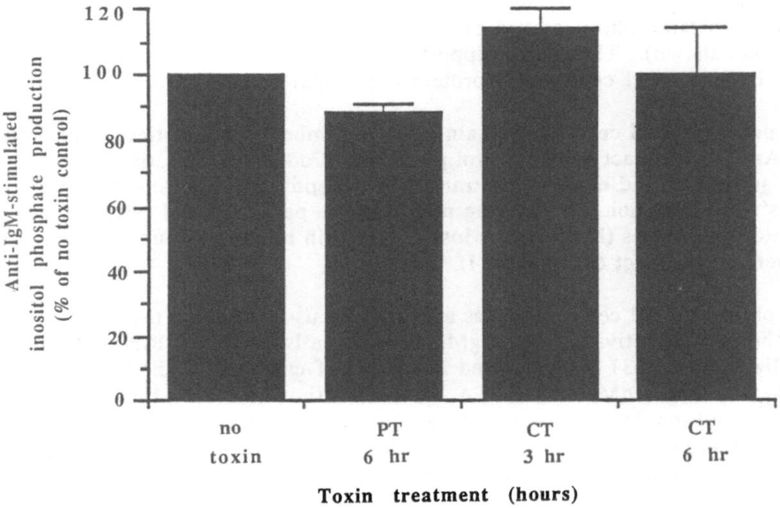

Figure 3. Pertussis toxin and cholera toxin do not block anti-IgM-stimulated production of inositol phosphates. Intact WEHI-231 cells were treated with 100 ng/ml of pertussis toxin (PT) or cholera toxin (CT) for the indicated lengths of time before being incubated with 10 μg/ml anti-IgM for 10 minutes. The production of total inositol phosphates was determined and is expressed as a percent of the inositol phosphate production by cells that had not been exposed to toxins. Each bar is the average and range of two experiments.

Initial Characterization of the G Protein

Many different receptors activate the phosphoinositide signaling system. Recent evidence in a number of different cell types has demonstrated that G proteins couple these receptors to phospholipase C. An important question is whether all these receptors utilize the same G protein or whether cells possess multiple G proteins that couple receptors to phospholipase C. Having multiple G proteins that serve this purpose might allow independent regulation of signaling by different receptors.

One way to distinguish among G proteins is by their sensitivity to two bacterial toxins, cholera toxin and pertussis toxin. These toxins cause covalent modification (ADP-ribosylation) of different G proteins and disrupt their ability to interact with receptors. For example, cholera toxin modifies G_s, the G protein that activates adenylate cyclase while pertussis toxin modifies G_i, the G protein that inhibits adenylate cyclase. To characterize the G protein that couples mIgM to phospholipase C, we treated intact WEHI-231 cells with 100 ng/ml of either cholera toxin or pertussis toxin for 3-6 hours and then assayed the ability of anti-IgM to stimulate inositol phosphate production. Figure 3 shows that none of these treatments blocked signaling by mIgM. To test whether the toxins had actually modified the relevant G protein substrates, we isolated membranes from the treated cells and treated them in vitro with the corresponding toxin and ^{32}P-NAD. No further ADP-ribosylation of pertussis toxin or cholera toxins substrates was seen in cells that had been treated with toxins in vivo[25]. Thus, under conditions in which all the major pertussis toxin and cholera toxin substrates had been modified, signaling by mIgM was unaffected. Therefore the G protein that couples mIgM to phospholipase C is one that is insensitive to both pertussis and cholera toxins. A number of other receptors that activate phospholipase C also utilize toxin-insensitive G proteins. This class of receptors includes the receptors for thyrotropin releasing hormone[26] and vasopressin[27]. In contrast, several receptors that activate phospholipase C utilize a G protein that is sensitive to pertussis toxin. Stimulation of inositol phosphate production by the neutrophil receptor for chemotactic peptides[28] as well as the receptor for angiotensin II[29] is blocked by pertussis toxin. Thus, by the criterion of toxin sensitivity, there appears to be at least two different G proteins that couple receptors to phospholipase C. Membrane Ig utilizes the one that is resistant to both pertussis and cholera toxins.

Regulation of Signaling by mIgM

Since signaling by mIgM is a crucial event in B cell activation, it is not surprising that this process is regulated by other agents that act on B cells. One documented example of such regulation involves the Fc receptor for IgG (FcR II) which inhibits mIgM-triggered PIP_2 breakdown if crosslinked to mIgM[22]. This inhibition appears to manifest itself at the interaction of mIgM with the G protein.

A second type of regulation of mIgM-triggered PIP_2 hydrolysis is mediated by protein kinase C[30,31]. We have shown that agents that activate protein kinase C inhibit mIgM-mediated PIP_2 breakdown in WEHI-231 cells. The biologically active phorbol esters, phorbol dibutyrate (PdBu), 4ß-phorbol didecanoate and phorbol myristate acetate (PMA), all inhibited the generation of inositol phosphates (InsP, $InsP_2$, $InsP_3$, and $InsP_4$) in response to the crosslinking of mIgM (Table II and ref. 30). In contrast, the inactive phorbol ester, 4α-phorbol didecanoate, did not block signaling by mIgM[30]. Phorbol esters mimic the action of the natural activator of protein kinase C, diacylglycerol (DG). As expected, treatment of WEHI-231 cells with a synthetic DG, dioctanoylglycerol (diC_8), also inhibited the ability of anti-IgM to stimulate the production of inositol phosphates (Table III). This decrease in inositol phosphate production reflected an inhibition of PIP_2 breakdown, rather than an increased rate of dephosphorylation of the inositol phosphates, since production of DG, the other second messenger derived from PIP_2 was also blocked by treating WEHI-231 cells with phorbol esters[30]. The production of DG was determined indirectly, by measuring the production of phosphatidic acid, the phosphorylated derivative of DG. Phorbol esters and diC_8 also blocked the ability of anti-IgM to cause increases in cytoplasmic calcium in WEHI-231 cells, consistent with the evidence that the rise in intracellular calcium is due to the calcium-mobilizing action of $InsP_3$. Thus, activation of protein kinase C in WEHI-231 cells blocks the production of all PIP_2-derived second messengers, apparently by preventing mIgM-mediated activation of phospholipase C.

Table 2. Phorbol Dibutyrate Blocks Anti-IgM-Stimulated Inositol Phosphate Production.

Additions[a]		^{3}H-inositol phosphates (cpm)			
anti-IgM	PdBu	InsP	$InsP_2$	$InsP_3$	$InsP_4$
-	-	97 ± 3	128 ± 4	59 ± 29	45 ± 5
+	-	574 ± 16	646 ± 36	532 ± 26	112 ± 2
+	+	110 ± 12	174 ± 16	134 ± 14	52 ± 6
		(97%)[b]	(92%)	(84%)	(90%)

a ^{3}H-inositol-labelled WEHI-231 cells were incubated with 1 μM phorbol dibutyrate (PdBu) or buffer for 10 minutes before addition of 10 μg/ml anti-IgM or PBS.

b Per cent inhibition of anti-IgM-stimulated inositol phosphate production. Reprinted from Gold and DeFranco[30] by permission of the Journal of Immunology.

Protein kinase C could inhibit mIgM-mediated PIP_2 breakdown by phosphorylating either mIgM, the G protein or phospholipase C. The mIgM is not a likely site for protein kinase C action because its cytoplasmic tail consists of only 3 amino acid residues, lysyl-valyl-lysine, none of which are normally substrates for serine/threonine kinases such as protein kinase C. In addition, we have found that short-term treatment of WEHI-231 cells with phorbol esters did not decrease the expression of mIgM[30]. Phorbol esters do cause rapid down regulation of other cell surface molecules such as the Ti/T3 complex and the transferrin receptor, but this is not the case with mIgM in WEHI-231 cells.

Two possibilities remained. Protein kinase C activation could inhibit either the G protein or the phospholipase C. To distinguish between these possibilites, we employed a broken cell system in which phospholipase C can be activated either directly with calcium or via the G protein upon addition of aluminum fluoride or stable GTP analogues. In this system, ^{3}H-inositol-labelled WEHI-231 cells are broken either by hypotonic swelling followed by homogenization with a Dounce homogenizer or by sonication. Incubation of this homogenate with GTPγS, aluminum fluoride or 1 mM calcium stimulated the production of inositol phosphates (Table IV). Addition of anti-IgM antibodies in the absence of added guanine nucleotide or in the presence of GTP or GTPγS did not stimulate the production of inositol phosphates (data not shown). Similar results were obtained with membranes pelleted from the homogenate. These results were different than what was seen with permeabilized WEHI-231 cells where GTPγS caused little inositol phosphate production by itself but potentiated the effects of anti-IgM antibodies. In these homogenates and membrane preparations, the G protein could be fully activated by GTPγS without stimulation by anti-IgM. At present, we do not understand why the two systems differ. Inclusion of protease inhibitors during homogenization had no effect suggesting that proteolysis is not responsible. Nevertheless, we could employ this broken cell system to assess G protein function independently of mIgM function.

Using this broken cell system, we found that phorbol esters inhibited both G protein-mediated and calcium-stimulated activation of phospholipase C. When intact WEHI-231 cells were treated with 1 μM PMA for 15 minutes at 37°C before being

Table 3. DiC_8 Inhibits Anti-IgM-Stimulated Inositol Phosphate Production.

diC_8 (μM)[a]	% inhibition of InsP3 + InsP4 production[b]	n[c]
3	18 ± 9	3
10	35 ± 13	5
30	46 ± 15	5
100	78 ± 7	4

a ^{3}H-inositol-labelled WEHI-231 cells were incubated with diC_8 for 10 minutes before the addition of 10 μg/ml anti-IgM.

b Per cent inhibition of anti-IgM-stimulated production of $InsP_3$ + $InsP_4$; mean and standard deviation for multiple experiments.

c Number of experiments in which the indicated concentration of diC_8 was tested. Reprinted from Gold and DeFranco[30] by permission of the Journal of Immunology.

Table 4. Inositol Phosphate Production by Broken WEHI-231 Cells.[a]

Stimulus	Total inositol phosphates (cpm)
None	14 ± 48
GTPγS, 100 μM	1484 ± 40
GTPγS, 3 μM	718 ± 104
NaF, 20 mM	2839 ± 143
NaF, 10 mM	2104 ± 39
NaF, 3 mM	802 ± 15
Ca^{2+}, 1 mM	2362 ± 58

[a] ^{3}H-inositol-labelled WEHI-231 cells were broken by hypotonic swelling followed by homogenization using a Dounce homogenizer. The broken cells were incubated with the indicated stimuli for 10 minutes before the reactions were stopped and the production of inositol phosphates was determined. The data represent the average and range of duplicate samples. Samples receiving NaF also included 10 μM AlC_{13}.

homogenized, the ability of GTPγS to stimulate inositol phosphate production was inhibited by 75-85% relative to homogenates of untreated cells. Stimulation of inositol phosphate production by aluminum fluoride was also inhibited by 50-70%, depending on the experiment (Gold and DeFranco, manuscript in preparation). These results demonstrate that the G protein is no longer able to stimulate phosphoipase C after activation of protein kinase C. However, this could be due to an effect on the phospholipase rather than on the G protein. Interestingly, PMA reduced the ability of 1 mM calcium to activate phospholipase C, by approximately 40%. Similar results were obtained when the cells were treated with 100 μM diC_8 (Gold and DeFranco, manuscript in preparation). Thus, phorbol esters strongly inhibit the G protein-phospholipase C interaction and, to a lesser extent, inhibit calcium activation of the enzyme. At least two explanations for these results are possible. Protein kinase C could phosphorylate phospholipase C, resulting in a change in the enzyme (e.g., conformation, localization, etc.) that strongly inhibits its interaction with the G protein and also partially reduces the ability of calcium to activate the enzyme. Alternatively, protein kinase C could phosphorylate both the G protein and phospholipase C. In order to distinguish between these possibilities, it will be necessary to demonstrate phosphorylation of the components and to reconstitute the system with components from phorbol ester-treated and control cells.

What is the significance of protein kinase C regulation of signaling by mIgM? One role of this process would be as a feedback inhibition mechanism that limits the magnitude and duration of signaling by mIgM. When crosslinking mIgM causes PIP_2 breakdown, DG is produced. This DG would activate protein kinase C which in turn would have a negative effect on mIgM-mediated PIP_2 breakdown. Mizuguchi et al.[32] demonstrated that this sort of feedback mechanism occurs in the BAL17 B lymphoma cell line. They found that the anti-IgM-stimulated increase in cytoplasmic calcium was greater when protein kinase C activation was blocked by the inhibitor H-7. Activation or inhibition of protein kinase C may also be a mechanism by which exogenous agents such as lymphokines could regulate signaling by mIgM Production of DG by means other than breakdown of PIP_2 would activate protein kinase C and presumably inhibit signaling by mIgM. There is now evidence for receptor-stimulated breakdown of phosphatidylcholine which would generate DG[33]. It is of interest to see if this pathway is operative in B cells and if so, whether it inhibits signaling by mIgM as we would predict. Alternatively, agents that inhibit protein kinase C might be expected to act like H-7 and potentiate signaling by mIgM. It has recently been reported that sphingosine and lyso-sphingolipids can inhibit protein kinase C[34]. At this point, it is unclear whether receptor activation can modulate the generation of these compounds. Thus protein kinase C may be an important locus by which mIgM-mediated signaling is modulated.

SUMMARY

The antigen receptors on B lymphocytes, membrane forms of immunoglobulins, transduce signals regulating B cell growth and differentiation by activating a phosphoinositide-specific phospholipase C. In this report, we describe our recent work aimed at understanding this process in greater detail. We have shown that a GTP-binding component is a necessary cofactor in the stimulation of phospholipase C by mIgM. This component has a number of properties in common with the G protein family of receptor-effector coupling components seen in the adenylate cyclase and other signaling systems. For example, analogues of GTP that cannot be hydrolyzed stimulated mIgM-triggered phosphoinositide breakdown, and an analogue of GDP that cannot be converted to GTP inhibited the reactions. Furthermore, aluminum fluoride, which activates known G proteins, also stimulates phosphoinositide breakdown. The G protein that appears to link mIgM to phospholipase C is not one of the well characterized G proteins involved in the regulation of adenylate cyclase or cGMP phosphodiesterase (G_s, G_i, and transducin), as judged by its insensitivity to two bacterial toxins that modify these G proteins, cholera toxin and pertussis toxin. Interestingly, analysis of pertussis toxin sensitivity indicates that there are at least 2 distinct G proteins that couple receptors to phospholipase C. For example, the G protein required for chemotactic peptide receptor signaling in neutrophils is sensitive to pertussis toxin, in contrast to the phosphoinositide signaling G protein in B cells.

We have also begun to explore the mechanisms by which mIgM signal transduction can be modulated. Stimulation of protein kinase C with phorbol esters or synthetic DG was found to inhibit mIgM-triggered phosphoinositide breakdown. This regulation probably represents a feedback inhibition that would occur with DG produced by phosphoinositide breakdown. Alternatively, there appear to be other signaling pathways that generate DG[33], and they could possibly inhibit phosphoinositide breakdown via protein kinase C. This could be an important locus of regulation during B cell activation. For example, other signals could increase or decrease the potency of this feedback inhibition, and thereby adjust the sensitivity of the B cell to antigen. Alternatively, other agents could stimulate protein kinase C directly, or could stimulate another protein kinase which can do the same thing in this regard, and thereby make the B cell insensitive to antigen by preventing antigen receptor signaling.

The mechanism by which protein kinase C inhibits mIgM-signal transduction is beginning to be understood. The stimulation of phospholipase C by agents that work by directly acting on the G protein, non-hydrolyzable analogues of GTP and aluminum fluoride, is blocked substantially by pretreatment of the cells with phorbol diesters. Stimulation of the phospholipase C by high concentrations of calcium, which probably does not require the G protein, is blocked to a lesser, but still significant degree. The simplest explanation of these results is that protein kinase C may phosphorylate phospholipase C making it unable to interact with the G protein, and only partially able to hydrolyze its substrate in the presence of 1 mM Ca^{2+}. This hypothesis is currently being tested. Inhibition by this mechanism has the effect of uncoupling all receptors that induce phosphoinositide breakdown. Interestingly, the inhibition of antigen receptor signaling induced by the Fc receptor appears to act earlier, at the receptor or receptor/G protein interaction, leaving open the possibility that other receptors that induce phosphoinositide breakdown could be unaffected. Thus, two different sites of regulation of antigen receptor signal transduction have been identified to date in B cells. The relevance of these two mechanisms for the different modes of B cell activation remains to be elucidated.

ACKNOWLEDGEMENTS

This work was supported by Grant AI-20038 from the National Institutes of Health. M.R.G. was an Arthritis Foundation postdoctoral fellow. We thank our colleagues who contributed to this work, including Dr. J.P. Jakway and K.A. Fahey.

REFERENCES

1. G.J.V. Nossal, Cellular mechanisms of immunologic tolerance, Ann. Rev. Immunol. 1:33 (1983).
2. D.C. Parker, J.J. Fothergill, and D.C. Wadsworth, B lymphocyte activation by insoluble anti-immunoglobulin: Induction of immunoglobulin secretion by a T cell-dependent soluble factor, J. Immunol. 123:931 (1979).
3. A.L. DeFranco, Molecular aspects of B lymphocyte activation, Ann. Rev. Cell Biol. 3:143 (1987).
4. B.L. Pike, A.W. Boyd, and G.J.V. Nossal, Clonal anergy: the universally anergic B lymphocyte, Proc. Natl. Acad. Sci. USA 79:2013 (1982).
5. K.L. Rock, B. Benacerraf, and A.K. Abbas, Antigen presentation by hapten-specific B lymphocytes. I. Role of surface immunoglobulin receptors, J. Exp. Med. 160:1102 (1984).
6. H.-P. Tony and D.C. Parker, Major histocompatability complex-restricted polyclonal B cell responses resulting from helper T cell recognition of anti-immunoglobulin presented by small B lymphocytes, J. Exp. Med. 161:223 (1985).
7. A. Lanzavecchia, Antigen-specific interaction between T and B cells, Nature 314:537 (1985).
8. G. Moller, Effects of anti-immunoglobulin sera on B lymphocyte function, Immunol. Rev. 52:1 (1980).
9. M.K. Bijsterbosch, C.J. Meade, G.A. Turner, and G.G.B. Klaus, B lymphocyte receptors and polyphosphoinositide degradation, Cell 41:999 (1985).
10. M.J. Berridge, Inositol trisphosphate and diacylglycerol: two interacting second messengers, Ann. Rev. Biochem. 56:159 (1987).
11. J. Braun, R. Sha'afi, and E.R. Unanue, Crosslinking by ligands to surface immunoglobulin triggers mobilization of intracellular Ca^{2+} in B lymphocytes, J. Cell Biol. 82:755 (1979).
12. T. Pozzan, P. Arslan, R.Y. Tsien, and T.J. Rink, Anti-immunoglobulin, cytoplasmic free calcium, and capping in B lymphocytes, J. Cell Biol. 94:335 (1982).
13. K.A. Fahey and A.L. DeFranco, Crosslinking membrane IgM induces production of inositol trisphosphate and inositol tetrakisphosphate in WEHI-231 B lymphoma cells, J. Immunol. 138:3935 (1987).
14. J.G. Monroe and M.J. Kass, Molecular events in B cell activation I. Signals required to stimulate G_0 to G_1 transition of resting B lymphocytes, J. Immunol. 135:1674 (1985).
15. J.T. Ransom and J.C. Cambier, B cell activation VII. Independent and synergistic effects of mobilized calcium and diacylglycerol on membrane potential and I-A expression, J. Immunol. 136:66 (1986).
16. T.L. Rothstein, T.R. Baeker, R.A. Miller, and D.L. Kolber, Stimulation of murine B cells by the combination of calcium ionophore plus phorbol ester, Cell. Immunol. 102:364 (1986).
17. G.G.B. Klaus, A. O'Garra, M.K. Bijsterbosch, and M. Holman, Activation and proliferation signals in mouse B cells VIII. Induction of DNA synthesis in B cells by a combination of calcium ionophore and phorbol myristate acetate, Eur. J. Immunol. 16:92 (1986).
18. P. Ralph, Functional subsets of murine and human B lymphocyte cell lines, Immunol. Rev. 48:107 (1979).
19. A.W. Boyd and J.S. Schrader, The regulation of growth and differentiation of a murine B cell lymphoma II. The inhibition of WEHI-231 by anti-immunoglobulin antibodies, J. Immunol. 126:2466 (1981).
20. R.F. Irvine and R.M. Moor, Micro-injection of inositol 1,3,4,5-tetrakisphosphate activates sea urchin eggs by a mechanism dependent on external Ca^{2+}, Biochem. J. 240:917 (1986).

21. A.P. Morris, D.V. Gallacher, R.F. Irvine, and O.H. Peterson, Synergism of inositol trisphosphate and tetrakisphosphate in activating Ca^{2+}-dependent K^+ channels, Nature 330:653 (1987).
22. M.K. Bijsterbosch and G.G.B. Klaus, Crosslinking of surface immunoglobulin and Fc receptors on B lymphocytes inhibits stimulation of inostiol phospholipid breakdown via the antigen receptor, J. Exp. Med. 162:1825 (1985).
23. L. Stryer and H.R. Bourne, G-proteins: a family of signal transducers, Ann. Rev. Cell Biol. 2:391 (1986).
24. A.G. Gilman, G proteins: transducers of receptor-generated signals, Ann. Rev. Biochem. 56:615 (1987).
25. M.R. Gold, J.P. Jakway, and A.L. DeFranco, Involvement of a guanine nucleotide-binding component in membrane IgM-stimulated phosphoinositide breakdown, J. Immunol. 139:3604 (1987).
26. T.F.J. Martin, D.O. Lucas, S.M. Bajjalieh, and J.A. Kowalchyk, Thyrotropin-releasing hormone activates a Ca^{2+}-dependent polyphosphoinositide phosphodiesterase in permeable GH3 cell. GTPγS potentiation by a cholera and pertussis toxin-insensitive mechanism, J. Biol. Chem. 261:2918 (1986).
27. R.J. Uhing, V. Prpic, H. Jiang, and J.H. Exton, Hormone-stimulated polyphosphoinositide breakdown in rat liver plasma membranes. Roles of guanine nucleotides and calcium, J. Biol. Chem. 261:2140 (1986).
28. C.D. Smith, B.C. Lane, I.Kusaka, M.W. Verghese, and R. Snyderman, Chemoattractant receptor-induced hydrolysis of phosphatidylinositol 4,5-bisphosphate in human polymorphonuclear leukocyte membranes. Requirement for a guanine nucleotide regulatory protein, J. Biol. Chem. 260:5875 (1985).
29. J. Pfeilschifter and C. Bauer, Pertussis toxin abolishes angiotensin II-induced phosphoinositide hydrolysis and prostaglandin synthesis in rat renal mesangial cells, Biochem. J. 236:289 (1986).
30. M.R. Gold and A.L. DeFranco, Phorbol esters and dioctanoylglycerol block anti-IgM-stimulated phosphoinositide hydrolysis in the murine B cell lymphoma WEHI-231, J. Immunol. 138:868 (1987).
31. J. Mizuguchi, M.A. Beaven, J. Hu Li, and W.E. Paul, Phorbol myristate acetate inhibits anti-IgM-mediated signaling in resting B cells, Proc. Natl. Acad. Sci. USA 83:815 (1986).
32. J. Mizuguchi, J. Yong-Yong, H. Nakabayaschi, K.-P. Huang, M.A. Beaven, T. Chused, and W.E. Paul, Protein kinase C activation blocks anti-IgM-mediated signaling in BAL17 lymphoma cells, J. Immunol. 139:1054 (1987)
33. J.M. Besterman, V. Duronio, and P. Cuatrecasas, Rapid formation of diacylglycerol from phasphatidylcholine: A pathway for generation of second messengers, Proc. Natl. Acad. Sci. USA 83:6785 (1986).
34. Y.A. Hannun, C.R. Loomis, A.H. Merrill, Jr., and R.M. Bell, Sphingosine inhibition of protein kinase C activity and of phorbol dibutyrate binding in vitro in human platelets, J. Biol. Chem. 261:12604 (1986).

VOLTAGE-SENSITIVE ION CHANNELS IN HUMAN B LYMPHOCYTES

Jeffrey B. Sutro, Bharathi S. Vayuvegula*, Sudhir Gupta*, and Michael D. Cahalan

Department of Physiology and Biophysics
and Division of Basic and Clinical Immunology
Department of Medicine (*)
University of California
Irvine, CA 92717

INTRODUCTION

Ion channels are protein pores that provide for the rapid movement of ions across cell membranes. Such channels control the transmembrane flow of ions by opening or closing in response to appropriate stimuli (a property referred to as gating) and by allowing only specific types of ions to pass through (a property referred to as selectivity). Although ion channels have been studied in nerve and muscle for many years (see 1 for a review), it is only since the development of the patch-clamp technique (2) that they have been detected in a variety of other tissues and systems. In the immune system such diverse cell types as T lymphocytes, B lymphocytes, macrophages, neutrophils, hybridomas, and natural killer cells express an assortment of channels (reviewed in 3).

Several studies on human and murine T lymphocytes have detected the presence of voltage-activated K^+ channels (Table 1) that must be functional in order for the cells to respond to mitogenic stimuli (4-7). In T lymphocytes, three types of K^+ channels have been detected based upon kinetic properties of gating, single channel conductance, and pharmacological specificity, and these three channel types are distributed in a subset-specific manner (8-10). Type *n* K^+ channels are the most commonly found variety, predominating in human T cells, rapidly proliferating immature murine thymocyte subsets, and in activated murine T cells (4-6, 8, 9). Types *n*' and *l* channels occur normally in murine T cells expressing cell-surface markers characteristic of the suppressor/cytotoxic phenotype, i.e., $CD4^-$ $CD8^+$ cells from thymus or spleen (10). Type *l* channels also are abundantly expressed in abnormally proliferating T cells from mice homozygous for the lpr or gld gene loci (11, 12). The diversity and pattern of K^+ channel expression are reviewed elsewhere (13).

Recently such studies have been extended to murine B lymphocytes (14, 15) which contain voltage-activated K^+ channels similar to those referred to as type "*n*" (8, 10) in murine T lymphocytes (Table 1). Resting BALB/c splenic B lymphocytes are small, with diameters ranging from 5 μm to 7 μm, but when treated with lipopolysaccharide (LPS) for 24 hrs. or longer they can enlarge (diameters of 8-13 μm), progress through DNA synthesis, and differentiate to the antibody-secreting stage of B-cell differentiation. In the resting stage murine B cells have an average of about 23 channels per cell.

When murine B cells enlarge in response to LPS stimulation they up-regulate the number of K^+ channels per cell, producing a 4-fold increase in the mean number of K^+ channels per unit membrane area (channel density). On average, a 10 µm diameter cell would have about 260 channels. Increased channel density following LPS treatment is closely associated with increased cell size; almost 95% of enlarged B cells have increased channel densities, while the mean channel density of LPS-treated cells that are not enlarged is the same as that for untreated cells. K-channel density was found to be independent of the length of time that the cell was exposed to the mitogen.

As a first step in assessing the functional significance of the K^+ channels in murine B lymphocytes we employed pharmacological probes (15, 16, manuscript in preparation). K^+ channels in murine B cells can be blocked by pharmacological agents such as verapamil ($K_{1/2}$ = 10 µM), cetiedel ($K_{1/2}$ = 20 µM), quinine ($K_{1/2}$ = 22 µM), 4-aminopyridine (4-AP) ($K_{1/2}$ = 300 µM), and tetraethylammonium (TEA) ($K_{1/2}$ = 10 mM). These same drugs block LPS-induced proliferation and antibody secretion, with a potency sequence corresponding to that for the block of K^+ channels. Since the mitogen-induced enlargement of B cells is not affected by these drugs, we hypothesized that functional K^+ channels are required for enlarged B lymphocytes to progress to the proliferating stage.

Murine T lymphocytes expressing CD4 but not CD8 (primarily helper T cells) have electrophysiological properties very similar to those of murine B lymphocytes (10, 15). Both cell types contain small numbers of type *n* K^+ channels when in the resting state, and respond to mitogenic stimuli by an increase in cell size in parallel with a dramatic increase of K^+ channel density (9, Table 1). In contrast, human T lymphocytes have densities of type *n* K^+ that are higher than those in murine T or B lymphocytes, whether resting or mitogen-activated. Human T cells enlarge in response to mitogenic stimuli, but do not increase their K^+ channel density (17, 18). Since murine T ($CD4^+$ cells) and B lymphocytes are so similar, it might be expected that the electrophysiology of human B lymphocytes would closely resemble that of human T lymphocytes. To test this supposition, we used the whole-cell patch-clamp technique to study human tonsillar B lymphocytes both before and after treatment with the mitogen *Staphylococcus aureus* Cowan I (SAC).

MATERIALS AND METHODS

Patch-clamp recording

A small glass micropipette (tip diameter ~1 µm), filled with an electrolyte solution, is positioned so that the tip comes into contact with the target cell. Since the tip has been fire-polished until smooth, a slight suction will cause a tight, high resistance (> 10^9 ohms) seal to form between the membrane and the pipette tip. Increased suction will then rupture the patch of membrane beneath the pipette tip, bringing the pipette solution into contact with the interior of the cell. The pipette can then be used as an electrode to apply a desired voltage across the cell's membrane, and to record the transmembrane currents elicited by the applied voltage. This is known as the whole-cell patch-clamp configuration (2), and was used in all the experiments reported here. Voltage stimuli were computer controlled, and output data were recorded on disk for future analysis. All voltages are reported as voltage inside the cell with the external solution grounded. Further details of the techniques are described elsewhere (8, 10, 19).

Solutions

External (bath) solutions used during experiments included:

Ringer (160 mM NaCl, 4.5 mM KCl, 2 mM $CaCl_2$, 1 mM $MgCl_2$, 5 mM HEPES buffer with pH adjusted to 7.4 with NaOH);

Table 1. Properties of Type *n* Potassium Channels in Lymphocytes

	Cell Type			
	HUMAN T	MOUSE T	HUMAN B	MOUSE B
K^+ channels per unactivated cell (6 um diameter) *	340	10	60	23
K^+ channels activated/cell (9 um diameter) *	820	430	420	210
unactivated K^+ channel density (channels/pF) *	280 ± 140	6	38 ± 20	14
activated K^+ channel density (channels/pF) *	300 ± 190	120	120 ± 30	56
increased membrane area after mitogen activation	~2.5 fold	~2 fold	~2 fold	~4.5 fold
single channel conductance (pS)	16 or 9	12	17	16
voltage at which 50% of channels open (mV)	-36	-36	-23 ± 7	-20 ± 6
inactivation time constant at +40 mV (msec)	~300 ± 120	110	140 ± 40	140 ± 52
channel closing time constant at -60 mV (msec)	~50 ± 20 •	49	53 ± 20	37 ± 10
sodium:potassium permeability ratio (P_{Na}/P_K) *	<0.01	0.02	0.02	0.02
channel blockers @	TEA, 4AP QUI, VER DIL, CTX	TEA, 4AP QUI, VER DIL, CET NIF	CTX	TEA, 4AP QUI, VER CET, NIT NIM, BAY
cells occasionally contain Na^+ channels	YES	YES	YES	NO
references	4-6,19,20	8,10,20	!	15

! This chapter
* Calculated from published data.
@ TEA=tetraethylammonium, 4AP=4-aminopyridine, QUI=quinine, VER=verapamil, DIL=diltiazem, CTX=charybdotoxin, CET=cetiedil, NIF=nifedipine, NIT=nitrendipine, NIM=mimodipine, BAY=BAY K 8644.

K^+ Ringer (160 mM KCl, 4.5 mM NaCl, 2 mM $CaCl_2$, 1 mM $MgCl_2$, 5 mM HEPES with pH adjusted to 7.4 with KOH).

The internal (pipette) solution used in these studies was KF (134 mM KF, 11 mM K_2EGTA, 1 mM $CaCl_2$, 2 mM $MgCl_2$, 5 mM HEPES with pH adjusted to 7.2 with KOH)

Cells

Human tonsillar B cells were grown in RPMI-1640 medium with 10% fetal calf serum with or without SAC Pansorbin (Calbiochem) at a final dilution of $1{:}10^{-5}$ from stock solution.

RESULTS AND DISCUSSION

Characterization of K^+ Channels in Human Tonsillar B Lymphocytes

As with most other types of lymphocytes, the predominant channel in human tonsillar B lymphocytes (Table 1) is a voltage-activated, type "*n*", K^+ channel (8). Figure 1A shows the K^+ currents evoked by a series of voltage steps from a holding potential of -80 mV to the indicated test voltages (all voltages measured inside the cell). At -80 mV K^+ channels are closed (the resting state), but they open within a few milliseconds at the test voltage, allowing K^+ ions to flow out of the cell, and produce an outward current (shown as an upward deflection). K^+ channels then progress into an "inactivated" (nonconducting) state, a process with time constant of from 100 to 200 msec. If the membrane potential is returned to -80 mV the channels will return to their resting state within 30 sec. At the more negative test voltages the K^+ channels open more slowly, and have a lower steady-state probability of opening. The voltage dependence of K^+ channel opening is illustrated in Figure 1B where the number of K^+ channels opening during each test pulse (calculated from the data in Figure 1A) is plotted vs. voltage.

Both the voltage dependence and the time course of channel gating illustrated in Figure 1 are typical of type *n* K^+ channels. To confirm that these channels are K^+ selective, we performed experiments like those shown in Figure 2. A brief initial voltage pulse to +30 mV opens a large proportion of the channels and the membrane potential is then stepped to the indicated test voltages. Currents measured at these test voltages are referred to as tail currents and decay toward zero as the channels close (Figure 2A). At the less negative voltages, the tail currents flow out of the cell, because the concentration of K^+ ions is high (160 mM) inside the cell, and lower (4.5 mM) outside the cell, and the K^+ ions tend to flow down their concentration gradient. However, negative membrane potentials tend to pull the positively charged K^+ ions into the cell, and if the test voltage is made negative enough the current will "reverse" and flow inward. The voltage where the tail current reverses (reversal potential) depends on the ionic selectivity of the channel and the concentrations of permeant ions to which the channel is exposed.

The reversal potential can be determined by extrapolating the tail currents back to the start of the test pulse, and plotting the extrapolated currents against voltage (Figure 2B). For the data in Figure 2 this procedure gives a reversal potential of -90 mV. When the external solution is changed to K^+ Ringer there is no K^+ concentration gradient across the membrane, so the reversal potential of a K^+-selective channel should be close to 0 mV. Experiments of this sort show that these channels are mainly permeant to K^+; the permeability to Na^+ calculated from such data is only 2% of the permeability to K^+. With a K^+ Ringer external solution the K^+ conductance is much larger than in Na^+ Ringer, as seen from the slope of the K^+ Ringer data in Figure 2B. Strong selectivity for K^+ over Na^+ and increased conductance in a high K^+ external solution are typical of type *n* K^+ channels (8, 19).

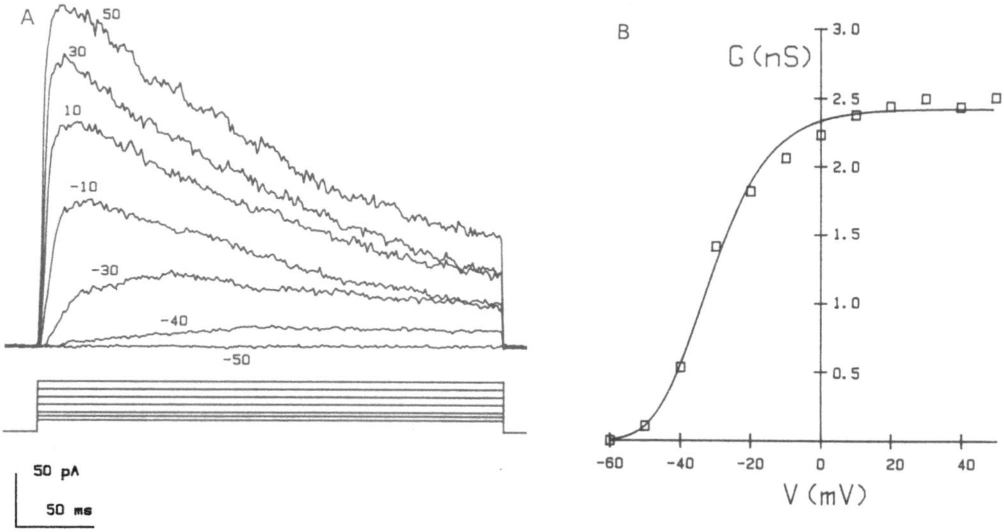

Figure 1. A. Potassium (K^+) currents evoked by voltage steps to the indicated membrane potentials in a human tonsillar B cell. B. Conductance-voltage relation for the same cell. Conductance, g_K (E), is computed from the measured peak current at each potential, divided by the electrical driving force, i.e., membrane potential minus K^+ equilibrium potential. The smooth curve represents a least-squares fit of the Boltzmann equation to the data points:

$$g_K (E) = g_{K\ max} / \{1 = \exp[(E_n - E)/k]\}^4,$$

where $g_{K\ max}$ represents the maximum K^+ conductance (proportional to the number of open channels), E_n is the characteristic membrane potential, a measure of where channels open, E is the membrane potential, and k is a slope factor, with the following parameters: $g_{K\ max}$ = 2.5 nS, E_n = -31 mV, and k = 10 mV.

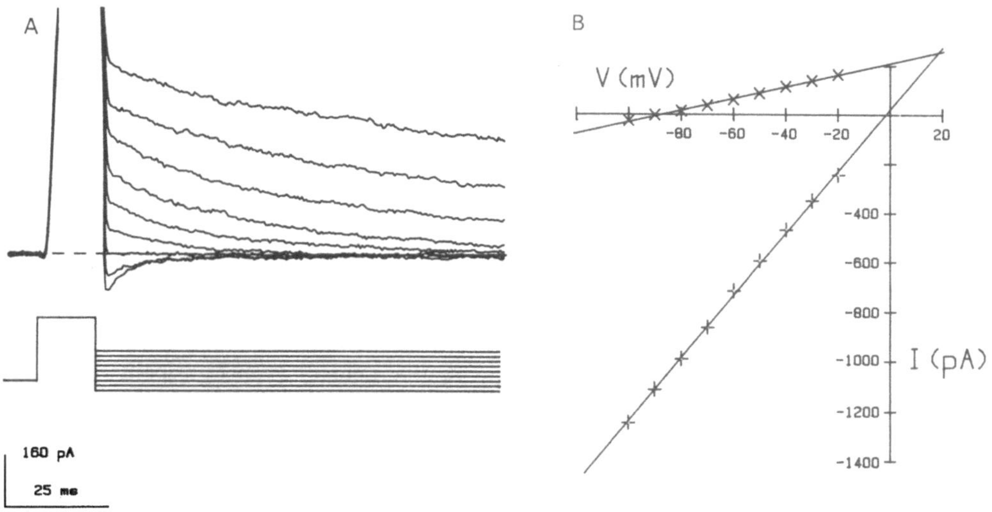

Figure 2. A. K^+ current transients corresponding to the closing of K^+ channels at various potentials. When the membrane potential is -90 mV, the current is near zero, indicating that this is the reversal potential for current through the K^+ channels. B. Instantaneous current-voltage relations in normal (X) and K^+ Ringer (+). The shift in reversal potential demonstrates that the channels are primarily permeable to K^+ ions.

In fact, by all the criteria that we have examined (Table 1), the K^+ channels in human B lymphocytes resemble type *n* K^+ channels. We have not yet studied the response of these K^+ channels to channel blocking agents, but it is very likely that their pharmacology is like that of other type *n* K^+ channels. Since verapamil, quinine, 4-AP, and TEA can block anti-IgM induced proliferation, with a potency sequence identical to that for the block of type *n* K^+ channels (16), we are confident that functional K^+ channels are required if human B cells are to enter the proliferating stage of mitogen-induced differentiation.

Single Channels

Single channel currents were recorded from several human B cells (Figure 3). If voltage pulses are applied to the cell at a rate of 1 Hz, most of the K^+ channels become inactivated and do not have sufficient time between pulses to return to the resting state. Thus, only a small number of channels open during each pulse and we can resolve individual channel openings, as illustrated by the top seven traces of Figure 3. Two sorts of channels were seen during pulses to +10 mV, one that was inward and another that was outward. In the bottom trace of Fig. 3, individual sweeps to +10 mV are averaged together to reconstruct the ensemble behavior of these channels.

The outward currents shown in Figure 3 are through K^+ channels, with a single channel conductance of 17 pS. Since the inward currents were observed less often than the outward currents, their identity is less certain. They have a reversal potential around +70 or +80 mV, suggesting that they are either Na^+ or Ca^{++} channels. We believe that they are Na^+ currents for the following reasons: 1) Their single channel conductance is around 17 pS, a value consistent with that of other Na^+ channels, but much larger than that expected for Ca^{++} channels with only 2 mM Ca^{++} in the external solution; 2) In one cell we observed macroscopic inward currents, and the rate at which they develop and decay is more rapid than that of known Ca^{++} currents. Averaged single-channel records show similar rapid rates of opening and inactivation. To establish conclusively the identity of the inward channels, it will be necessary to measure the ionic selectivity of these channels, and their response to tetrodotoxin (TTX), a highly specific Na^+ channel blocking agent.

Although Na^+ channels occur in a small fraction of both human and murine T lymphocytes, they are not present in murine B lymphocytes; finding them in human B lymphocytes is thus somewhat unexpected. So far, a functional significance of lymphocyte Na^+ channels has not been demonstrated. Since their occurrence is sporadic, they may define some specialized lymphocyte sub-population whose function has not yet been discovered. Alternatively, lymphocyte Na^+ channels may be necessary only in unusual circumstances.

Response to Mitogenic Activation by SAC

Untreated human tonsillar B cells that we examined had diameters of 6 to 7 μm, on average slightly larger than the murine B cells studied previously. They contained an average of 60 K^+ channels per cell (6 μm diameter), 2.5 times the channel density of murine B lymphocytes, but far less than the 340 channels found in a 6 μm human T lymphocyte. Following 4 to 6 days of treatment with SAC, some of the human B cells had enlarged, with diameters ranging up to 9 μm. This slight enlargement in response to mitogen activation is less than that of murine B cells, which enlarge dramatically (diameters of 8 to 13 μm).

Some human B cells responded to SAC treatment with an up-regulation of their K^+ channels to about 3 times the K^+ channel density measured in untreated cells (Figure 4). Other SAC-treated cells had K^+ channel densities similar to those seen in untreated cells. In contrast to murine B lymphocytes, where the increase in channel density is confined to enlarged cells, the up-regulation of K^+ channels in human B lymphocytes appears unrelated to changes in cell size (Figure 4). These differences between human and murine B cells could be due to the fact that the majority of human

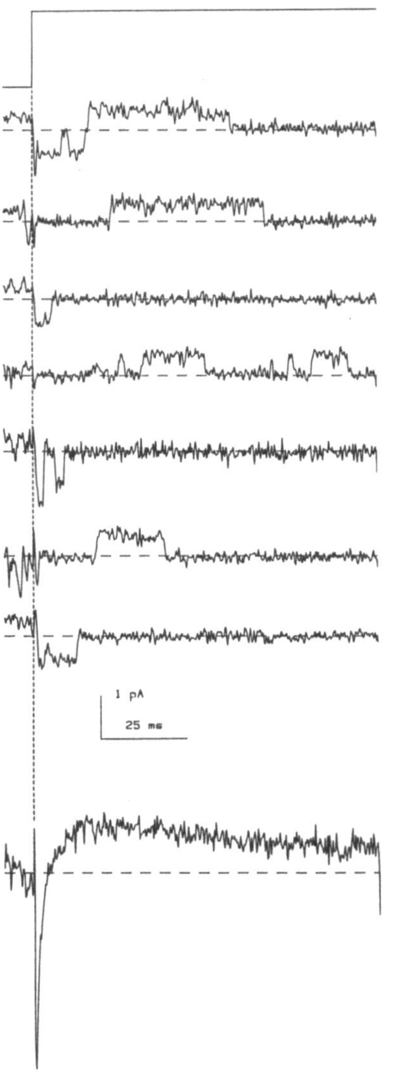

Figure 3. Each trace shows the current evoked by a 100 msec long test pulse to +10 mV, with the dotted vertical line drawn in to mark the start of the pulse, and the dashed horizontal line showing the zero current level. Single channel conductance was determined by measuring the single channel currents at each voltage, plotting them vs. voltage, and drawing a straight line through the data.

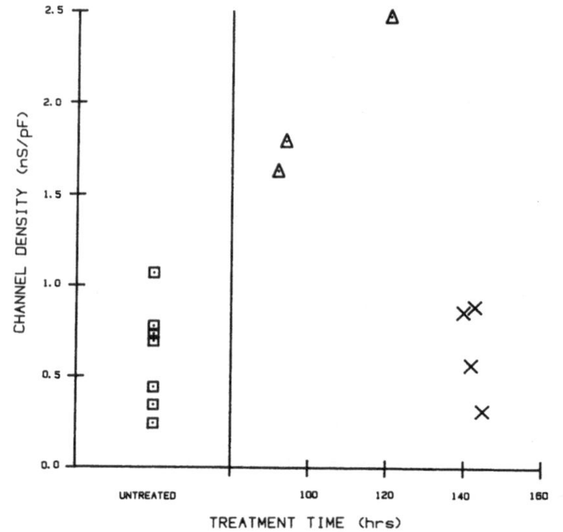

Figure 4. Density of K^+ channels in resting and activated human B cells. The channel density axis in units of nS/pF represents the maximum K conductance, $g_{K\ max}$, as computed in Figure 1, divided by the cell's capacitance, a measure of cell surface area determined electrically from the capacitative charging transient in response to a 10 mV voltage step. 1pF of capacitance corresponds to roughly 100 μm^2 of membrane surface area. Assuming a single channel conductance of 17 pS and a value for the specific membrane capacitance of 1 $\mu F/cm^2$, a channel density of $1/\mu m^2$ would correspondence to 1.69 nS/pF. Channel density is seen to increase by about 100 hrs. and then later decrease after activation.

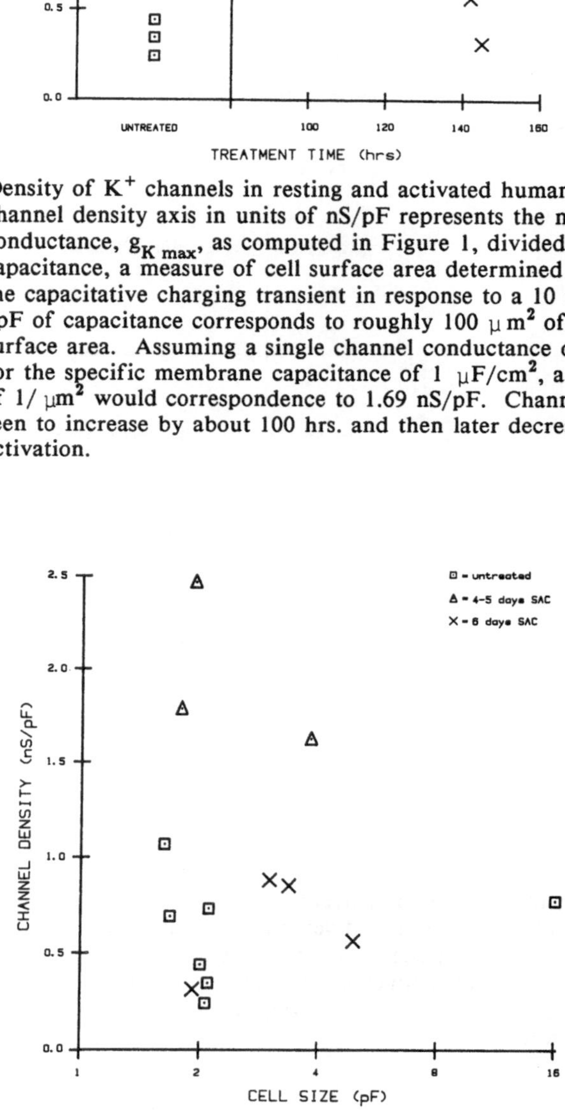

Figure 5. Channel density, as defined in the legend of Figure 4, plotted as a function of cell size. The highest densities were found 4-5 days after SAC treatment, but by 6 days channel density had declined, even though the cells were enlarged on average, relative to untreated cells.

tonsillar B cells are preactivated *in vivo*. Studies with resting B cells separated from preactivated B cells remain to be done.

There may, however, be a time-dependence to the K^+ channel density increase induced by SAC. Cells treated with SAC for 4 to 5 days (Figure 4) had increased K^+ channel densities, while cells treated with SAC for 6 days (Figure 4) had K^+ channel densities comparable to those of untreated cells. In Figure 5, the data from Figure 4 are plotted vs. time, to more clearly show the drop in channel density after 6 days of SAC treatment. Further experiments will be needed to confirm whether, in contrast to murine B lymphocytes, the mitogen-induced up-regulation of K^+ channels in human B lymphocytes is indeed time-limited.

SUMMARY

Human tonsillar B cells were found to contain type *n* K^+ channels, and have K^+ channel densities somewhere between those of murine B cells and those of human T cells. Unlike human T lymphocytes, some human B lymphocytes were able to increase K^+ channel density in response to mitogenic activation, but the increases were smaller than those observed in murine B lymphocytes. Some mitogen-stimulated human B cells increased in size, but, unlike murine B cells, cell size was not related to K^+ channel density. There may be a down-regulation of K^+ channel density in human B cells treated with SAC for 6 days, while no such effect occurs in murine B cells. A fraction of human B cells possess inward current channels (probably Na^+ channels) that are similar to channels sometimes seen in human T cells, but not seen in murine B cells.

ACKNOWLEDGMENTS

This study was supported by NIH grants NS-14609, AI26465 and GM-14514, and by a fellowship from the American Cancer Society to JBS.

REFERENCES

1. Hille, B: Ionic channels of excitable membranes. Sinauer Associates, Sunderland Mass. (1984).
2. Hamill OP, Marty A, Neher E, Sakmann B, Sigworth FJ: Improved patch-clamp techniques for high-resolution current recording from cells and cell-free membrane patches. Pfluegers Arch. 391: 85 (1981).
3. Cahalan MD, Chandy KG, DeCoursey TE, Gupta S, Lewis R, Sutro JB: Ion channels in T lymphocytes. In: Gupta S, Paul WE, and Fauci AS (Eds.), Mechanisms of Lymphocyte Activation and Immune Regulation. New York: Plenum Press, 1987.
4. DeCoursey TE, Chandy KG, Gupta S, Cahalan MD: Voltage-gated K^+ channels in human T lymphocytes: a role in mitogenesis? Nature 307: 465 (1984).
5. Chandy KG, DeCoursey TE, Cahalan MD, McLaughlin C, Gupta S: Voltage-gated K channels are required for T lymphocyte activation. J Exp Med 160: 369 (1984).
6. DeCoursey TE, Chandy KG, Gupta S, Cahalan MD: Voltage-dependent ion channels in T-lymphocytes. J Neuroimmunol 10: 71 (1985).
7. Lee SC, Sabath DE, Deutsch C, Prystowsky MB: Increased voltage-gated potassium conductance during interleukin 2-stimulated proliferation of a mouse helper T lymphocyte clone. J Cell Biol 102: 1200 (1986).
8. DeCoursey TE, Chandy KG, Gupta S, Cahalan MD: Two types of potassium channels in murine T lymphocytes. J Gen Physiol 89: 379 (1987).
9. DeCoursey TE, Chandy KG, Gupta S, Cahalan MD: Mitogen induction of ion channels in murine T lymphocytes. J Gen Physiol 89: 405 (1987).
10. Lewis RS and Cahalan MD. Subset-specific expression of potassium channels in developing murine T lymphocytes. Science 239: 771 (1988).

11. Chandy KG, DeCoursey TE, Fischbach M, Talal N, Cahalan MD, Gupta S: Altered K^+ channel expression in abnormal T lymphocytes from mice with the lpr gene mutation. Science 233: 1197 (1986).
12. Grissmer S, Cahalan MD, Chandy KG: Abundant expression of type *l* K^+ channels: a marker for lymphoproliferative diseases? J Immunol 141: 1137 (1988).
13. Lewis RS and Cahalan MD: The plasticity of ionic channels: parallels between the nervous and immune systems. Trends in Neuroscience 11: 214 (1988).
14. Choquet D, Sarthou P, Primi D, Cazenave PA and Korn H. Cyclic AMP-modulated potassium channels in murine B cells and their precursors. Science 235: 1211 (1987).
15. Sutro JB, Vayuvegula BS, Gupta S and Cahalan MD. Up-regulation of voltage-sensitive K^+ channels in mitogen-stimulated B lymphocytes. Biophysical Journal 53: 460a (1988).
16. Vayuvegula B, Gollapudi S, Gupta S: Inhibition of human B cell proliferation by ion channel blockers. In: Gupta S, Paul WE and Fauci AS (Eds.), Mechanisms of Lymphocyte Activation and Immune Regulation. New York: Plenum Press (1987), Advances in Experimental Medicine and Biology 213: 237 (1987).
17. Lee S, Krause D, Deutsch C: Increased voltage-gated K^+ conductance in T-lymphocytes stimulated with phorbol ester. J Physiol 372: 405 (1986).
19. Cahalan MD, Chandy KG, DeCoursey TE, Gupta S: A voltage-gated potassium channel in human T lymphocytes. J Physiol 358:197 (1985).
20. Sands SB, Lewis RS and Cahalan MD: Charybdotoxin blocks voltage-gated K^+ channels in T lymphocytes. Biophys J 53: 260a (1988).

INTERLEUKINS AND B LYMPHOCYTE ACTIVATION

INTERLEUKINS 4 AND 5: MECHANISMS OF ACTION

Eva Severinson, Hee-Bom Moon, Susanne Bergstedt-Lindqvist, Ulla Persson, Christoph Heusser and Janet Stavnezer

Dept. of Immunol., Stockholm Univ., and Dept. of Clin. Immunol., Karolinska Hospital, Stockholm, Sweden and Pharma Research, Ciba-Geigy Ltd., Basel, Switzerland and Dept. of Microbiol. and Mol. Biol., Univ. of Massachusetts Med. School, Worcester, MA, USA.

INTRODUCTION

Interleukins 4 and 5 are two recently described lymphokines, which exist both in mouse and man[1-5]. Biochemical analysis and molecular cloning have aided in determining their structure as well as their function. It has recently become clear that lymphokines in general are not selective for a certain cell type and that they often have a broad range of activities. Although information regarding these activities is emerging with a very high speed, it is still uncertain what is their primary role in vivo and in what way their synthesis and action are regulated.

SYNTHESIS OF IL 4 AND IL 5

So far, most studies of IL 4 and 5 have been made using T cell produced material. However, a thorough study of which cell types can produce these factors have not been done. Many T cell lines and tumours are known to produce IL 4 and 5, but most of the lines were pre-selected for another purpose.

We have performed a limiting dilution analysis of cells responding in mixed lymphocyte cultures (MLC) across a class II barrier and tested supernatants from individual cultures for interleukin 2 (IL 2) or IL 4 activity[6]. The former test was performed by measuring DNA synthesis in the T cell line CTLL. However, it has recently become clear that this assay can also detect IL 4[7,8]. As a test for IL 4, two assays were performed, the so called IgG1 induction assay[9,10], which measures an increase in the IgG1 isotype in lipopolysaccharide (LPS) stimulated cultures and co-stimulation of DNA synthesis with anti-Ig (the BSF-1 assay).

The data are shown in Table I. As shown, there are many clones which can support DNA synthesis in CTLL cells by their secreted product, whereas there are very few which were positive in the IL 4 assays[11]. It was difficult to determine the precursor freuqency for IL 4 secretors, since there were so few positives and since these mostly occurred when there were on the average less than one growing cell per culture. This latter phenomenon indicates that when cultures originate from several precursors, the IL 4 activity is not detected. Whether this is caused by suppression or over-growth by non-IL 4 secreting precursors is not known. By analysing cultures stemming from less than one precursor, a minimal estimate of 3% IL 4 precursors and 97% IL 2 precursors can be made among cells in this kind of MLC. An even lower figure, one out of 300 Con A

Table I. Frequency studies of cells from MLC stimulated across Ia: Assay for growth or secretion of TCGF, IgG1 inducing activity or BSF-1 activity.

Cell source cells	No. cells/well	No. wells with growing cells	Activity measured in supernatants: no of positive/ total no of growing cultures TCGF	IgG1 induction	BSF-1
2°MLC	1000	24/25	24/24	0/24	0/24
	300	24/24	24/24	0/24	0/24
	100	24/24	20/20	2/20	1/20
	30	13/24	10/10	0/10	0/10
	3	66/480	44/47	1/47	1/47
	1	20/480	14/17	0/17	1/17
3°MLC	1000	24/24	2/2	0/2	0/2
	300	24/24	2/2	0/2	0/2
	100	24/24	2/2	0/2	0/2
	30	24/24	2/2	0/2	0/2
	3	107/476	50/51	2/51	2/51
	1	76/480	50/51	2/51	2/51

Two-month-old B6.C-H-2^{bm12} (bm12) mice were used as donors of responding cells. These were stimulated with irradiated spleen cells from C57BL.10 (B10) mice in mixed lymphocyte cultures (MLC) or limiting dilutions, as described. Cloning was performed 4 days after the last stimulation. Scoring of cultures with growing cells was done on days 10-14. Aliquots of cells from selected wells were tested for secretion of lymphokines in a spot test as described. In short, cells were washed, resuspended in medium plus Con A, incubated in 37°C, 5 percent CO_2 for 24 h and supernatants collected after centrifugation. Ten percent of these supernatants were added to CTLL or Con A blasts for the T cell growth factor (TCGF) tests, to LPS containing spleen cell cultures for the IgG1 induction test or to $F(ab')_2$ anti-Ig containing splenic B cell cultures for the BSF-1 test, as described[10,11]. Reprinted with permission from[6].

activated cells make mRNA encoding IL 4, as detected in in situ hybridization[12]. It has been been suggested that there exist two populations of helper cells, one secreting IL 2 and gamma-interferon and the other secreting IL 4[13]. The authors of the report also found that certain antigens gave rise almost exclusively to one of the two populations. In another recent paper, the stimuli dictated whether IL-4 would be secreted or not[14]. It is not surprising that established T cell clones have a set pattern of lymphokine secretion. This, however, does not necessarily mean that T cells are committed before stimulation.

T CELLS CAN RESPOND TO IL 4 AND IL 5

As mentioned above, the T cell line CTLL can respond by increased DNA synthesis to IL 4. However, the cells do not grow in IL 4. On the other hand, Concanavalin A (Con A) stimulated primary T cells can be stimulated both to increased DNA synthesis and growth

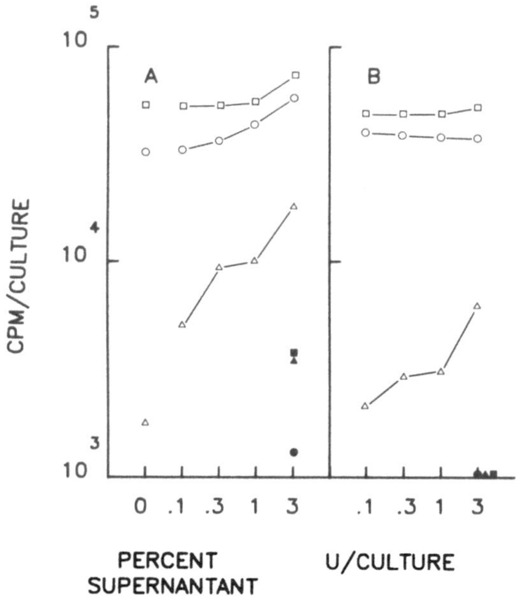

Fig. 1. Effect of IL 4 on T cell subpopulations. Nylon wool-purified cells were treated twice with anti-L3T4 (RL 172.4) or anti-Lyt-2 (3IM) antibodies plus complement. The nonfractionated cells (o, ●), the resulting Lyt-2^+ L3T4^- cells (△, ▲) or the L3T4^+ Lyt-2- cells (□, ■) were cultured alone (cpm/culture was 424, 620 and 746, respectively), or with Con A (open symbols). In addition different dilutions of IL 4-containing SN (H109) (A) or human rIL 2 (B) were added. Closed symbols correspond to cultures treated with the lymphokines alone. DNA synthesis was determined on day 3 by incubating with [3H]-thymidine for the last 24 h. Reprinted from[8].

by IL 4[8]. As shown in Figure 1, both CD 4 positive and CD 8 positive cells can respond to Con A plus IL 4.

It has been reported that among pre-existing T cell lines, those with helper phenotype repond to IL 4 better than those of killer phenotype[7]. Paradoxically, among primary T cells, the situation seems to be reverse[15]. However, in no case that we are aware of so far, does IL 4 stimulate a better proliferative response than IL 2 in T cells. In our minds, it would not be surprising if IL 2 would be the most important lymphokine for proliferation of mature T cells. On the other hand, it is possible that among differentiating thymocytes the situation is different, especially since the number of fetal thymocytes that produce mRNA encoding IL 4 has been found to be very high[12].

Whereas IL 4 stimulates T cells to proliferation, this is not the case with IL 5. In contrast, IL 5 induces functional IL 2 receptors on primary T cells, T cell lines as well as B cells[16].

IS IL 5 A B CELL LYMPHOKINE?

Mouse IL 5 has several effects on murine B cells, e.g. to cause an additive stimulation of DNA synthesis together with dextran sulphate, to stimulate the B cell tumor BCL_1 to increased DNA synthesis and IgM secretion and to substitute for T cells

Table II. Comparison between different IL 4 dependent assays.

Assay	U required for half-maximal activity	Stimulation index
Hyper-Ia expression	0.1	4
BSF-1 (anti-Ig mediated)	0.2	7
IgG1 induction	1	16
IgG3 reduction	9.5	22
TCGF assay (Con A blasts)	2.5	250

The indicated assays were performed using titration curves of the same batch of IL 4. The number of units required to obtain a half maximal response was calculated. 1 unit was defined as the concentration of IL 4 required to induce half maximal IgG1 induction in LPS cultures. Stimulation index was calculated by dividing the values obtained at maximal responses with background values.

in a secondary immune response in vitro. In human, there is a controversy as to the activity of IL 5 on B cells[5,17]. However, both in mouse and in man, there is a potent eosinophil differentiative activity of this interleukin. Sanderson and collegues have put forward the idea that the latter would be the main activity of IL 5[17]. Further studies are needed to resolve this point.

CONCENTRATION REQUIREMENTS OF IL 4

The amount of a lymphokine needed to stimulate a particular response in vitro can be a very important indication as to a possible in vivo significance. We made such a comparison of IL 4 in different assays[8]. For these experiments, the same batch of recombinant IL 4 or T cell produced IL 4, respectively was titrated in the various tests.

After the experiments were performed, the relative amount of IL 4 required to obtained a half-maximal response as well as the stimulation indeces were calculated (Table II). As shown, the capacity of IL 4 to induce an increased density of class II antigens on B cells was the most sensitive test, followed by the anti-Ig mediated BSF-1 test. These two assays were 10 and 5-fold more sensitive, respectively, than the IgG1 induction assay. The differences may reflect the relative in vivo importance of these activities of IL 4 on B cells and also the relative complexity of the tests. The IgG1 induction is measured after 5 days and involves a DNA recombination event, whereas class II induction is a 24 hour assay, not requirering DNA synthesis. The TCGF assay for IL 4 appears to be a relatively insensitive test, measured in this way. However, stimulation index as measured by the magnitude of the IL 4 induced response was high. IL 4 can also suppress the LPS induced IgG3 response. This activity is very insensitive, which may be related to a difficulty in observing a decrease of a high response as opposed to observing an increase of a low response.

REQUIREMENT FOR IgE INDUCTION WITH IL 4

It has become apparent in the last years that IL 4 production in parallel to the induction of IgG1 induce a switch to IgE secretion in LPS cultures[18]. It was of interest for us to to investigate this activity further.

We have made a long series of experiments in which we have tried to estimate the precursor frequencies for cells secreting various immunoglobulin classes in response to LPS or LPS plus IL 4[19]. In Table III, the results from two representative experiments are shown. Spleen cells from normal or nude mice were cultured in decreasing cell numbers in the presence of rat thymocytes passed over nylon wool as filler cells. On

Table III. Precursor frequency and clone size of IgM, IgG1, IgG3 and IgE secreting cells, stimulated by LPS or LPS plus IL 4.

		IgM		IgG1		IgG3		IgE	
		P.F.	C.S.	P.F.	C.S.	P.F.	C.S.	P.F.	C.S.
Exp. 1									
	LPS	1:65	(40)	1:1,900	(8.3)	1:290	17.5	N.T.	N.T.
	LPS+5% rIL 4	1:260	(15)	1:260	(6,3)	1:1,600	18.5	N.T.	N.T.
Exp. 2									
A	LPS	1:220	(93)	1:1,000	(1,6)	N.T.	N.T.	<<1:100.000	(75)
	LPS+3% rIL 4	1:225	(56)	1:176	(2,3)	N.T.	N.T.	1:200	(81)
B	LPS	1:14	(124)	1:360	(2,4)	N.T.	N.T.	<<1:100,000	(62)
	LPS+3% rIL 4	1:25	(83)	1:16	(4,6)	N.T.	N.T.	1:15	(108)

A limiting dilution analysis was performed using spleen cells from normal (Exp. 1 and 2A) or nude mice (Exp. 2B) cultured together with rat thymocytes as filler cells and LPS or LPS plus IL 4[19]. Culture supernatants were harvested on day 6 and analyzed for presence of Ig of different classes and subclasses using the ELISA.
P.F. = Precursor frequency
C.S. = Clone size.

day 6 after stimulation, the culture supernantants were removed and were tested for the presence of various Ig classes or subclasses in the enzyme linked immunosorbent assay (ELISA). For each cell concentration, the fraction of nonresponding cultures were calculated and the precursor frequency was estimated by extrapolation.

As shown in the table, the precursor frequency of IgM secretors decreased by the presence of IL 4 in some experiments but remained unchanged in another. The frequency of IgG3 secretors also decreased in the presence of IL 4. In contrast, the frequencies of IgG1 and IgE precursors increased dramatically in the presence of IL 4. The frequency of precursors for these two isotypes even surpassed the frequency of IgM precursors. In most experiments, the IgE frequency could not be determined in LPS cultures, since no positive cultures were found. For the same reason, the clone size could not be determined in these experiments. In experiments where a clone size could be calculated, no difference was found between responses in cultures containing LPS or LPS plus IL 4. By analysing individual cultures containing on the average less than one precursor per well, we could investigate to what extent each clone can produce more than one isotype. It was found that there existed clones that could secrete one, two or three isotypes in any combination. These results clearly indicate that the majority of the LPS reactive cells can switch to IgG1 and IgE, provided that IL 4 is also present. The results further indicate that B cells are not precommitted to switch to a particular isotype, but that they can switch to any isotype, depending on the stimuli.

Since certain clones could make both IgG1 and IgE, we wanted to determine whether cells first switched to IgG1 secretion and subsequently switched to secretion of IgE. If this was the case, one would expect that the appearance of the IgG1 isotype would preceed that of the IgE. As shown in Figure 2, the kinetics of appearance of these two isotypes are virtually identical, ruling out the possibility that all IgE secretors stem from IgG1 secretors. Next we investigated the effect of adding IL 4 in different concentrations to LPS cultures (Figure 3).

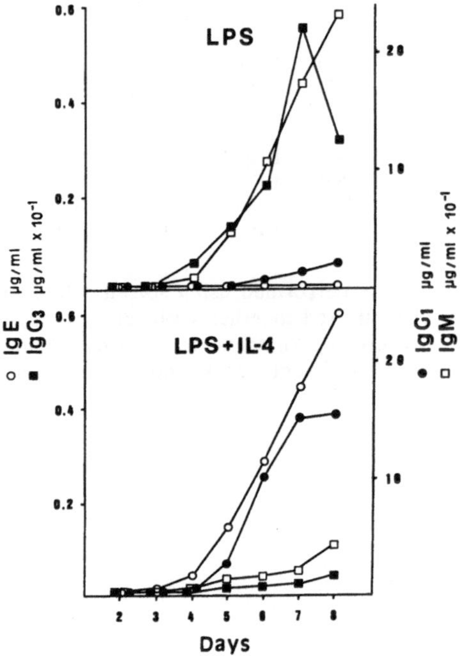

Fig. 2. Kinetics of the LPS or LPS plus IL 4 induced response. Supernatants from stimulated cultures were assayed in the ELISA at indicated times after onset of cultures.

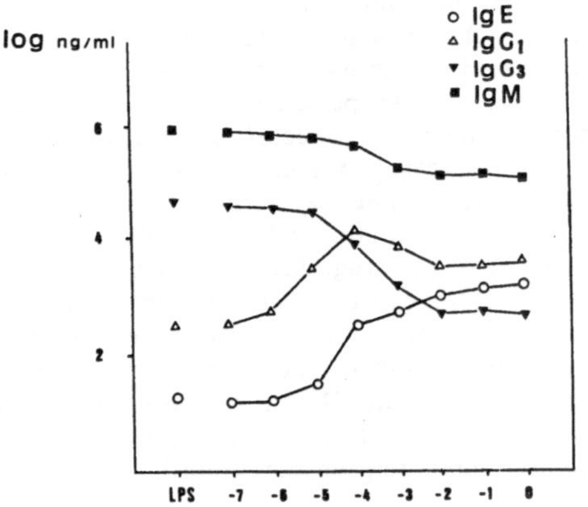

Fig. 3. The effect of IL 4 added at different concentrations to Ig responses. Cells stimulated with LPS alone or together with IL 4 at different doses. Responses were measured in the ELISA on day 6.

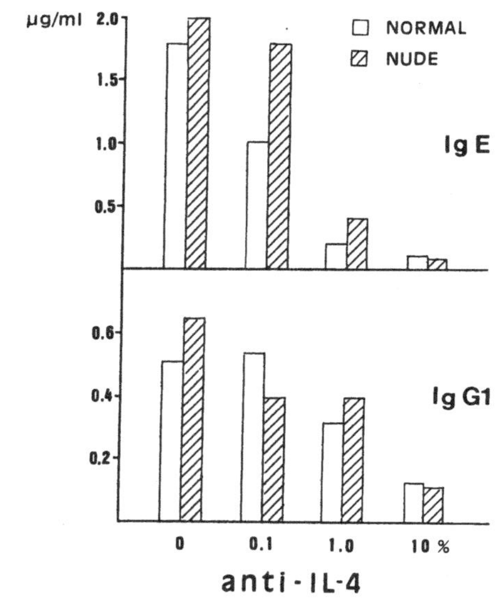

Fig. 4 Inhibition of IgE and IgG1 secretion by anti-IL 4. Spleen cells from normal or nude mice were cultured with LPS and IL 4 and different dilutions of supernatants from the anti-IL 4 hybridoma line (11B11). Responses were measured on day 6 in the ELISA.

The amount of IgM secreted after LPS stimulation was reduced by additions of high concentrations of IL 4, but the reduction of IgG3 was more marked, at the most hundred-fold. Induction of IgG1 secretion was evident at .003% IL 4 and reached a peak at .03%. On the other hand, IgE secretion was only detected at a 3-fold higher concentration and peaked at a 10-fold higher concentration than did IgG1.

Finkelman et al. recently published a report which has helped in clarifying the in vivo role of IL 4[20]. The parasite Nippostrongylus brasiliensis induces high IgE and IgG1 responses. It was shown that anti-IL 4 antibodies administered in vivo would inhibit the IgE response but not the IgG1 response. This might mean that IgG1 and IgE are differently regulated, or that IgG1 responses are more difficult to inhibit, since its response occurs at lower IL 4 concentrations, as seems evident in in vitro cultures. Indeed, as shown in Figure 4, in vitro addition of anti-IL 4 antibodies to cultures stimulated with LPS plus IL 4, inhibited both IgG1 and IgE responses although the latter were more profoundly inhibited. For example, at 1% anti-IL 4, the IgE responses were inhibited approximately 80%, whereas the IgG1 response was inhibited only 20-30%.

INDUCTION OF STERILE RNA TRANSCRIPTS BY IL 4

Stavnezer[21] and Alt[22] and their collegues have independently suggested a mechanism for starting V-D-J and S-S recombination, which mechanisms are involved in creation of the variable genes for heavy and light chains of Ig, and the switch event, respectively. The recombination events was suggested to be preceeded by an opening of the gene segments involved in the recombination by RNA transcription. To test this idea, we have investigated if RNA encoding γ and ε are synthesized prior to synthesis of the corresponding proteins. Normal mouse spleen cells were activated with LPS, IL 4 or the two stimuli together.

After 2 days, when no IgG1 or IgE protein is made as yet, RNA was extracted from the

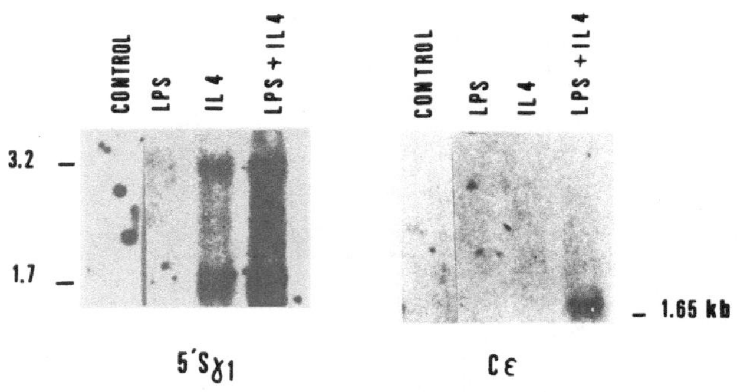

Fig. 5 Northern blotting of spleen cell RNA. Cells were stimulated with LPS, IL 4 or LPS plus IL 4 for 2 days, and total RNA was extracted from the cultured cells or from non-cultured spleen cells. Poly A^+ RNA was selected and 3 ug RNA were run per lane in agarose gels. The blotted nylon filters were hybridized with a 2 kb Hind III/Pst 1 fragment of the EH10 encoding the 5' $S\gamma_1$ region [23] or with a 2.9 kb Bam H1/Hind III segment encoding the germline $C\varepsilon_1$ gene[24].

cells and polyA+ RNA selected. Equal amounts of RNA from the cultured cells or RNA from normal spleen cells were thereafter analyzed by "Northern blotting". The result from one such experiment is shown in Figure 5. Two different probes were used, one encoding a segment immediately 5' of the $S\gamma_1$ region and the other encoding the $C\varepsilon$. As shown, there are two transcripts (3.2 and 1.7kb), encoding the 5'S $_1$ which are induced by IL 4 alone and stronger by LPS and IL 4 together. Furthermore, an RNA species of 1.65 kb, which is slightly shorter than the mature transcript, is stimulated by LPS and IL 4 together. Thus, these experiments support the hypothesis that S-S recombination is preceded by RNA transcription.

CONCLUDING REMARKS

IL 4 and IL 5 are both multifunctional lymohokines, with activities on B cells, T cells as well as on non-lymphoid cells. Although certain aspects of these responses are becoming clear, we probably have to investigate each type of response in much more detail, before we get a clear idea of their primary role in vivo.

ACKNOWLEDGEMENTS

We wish to thank Ms Lena Berggren for expert technical help and Ms Gunilla Tillinger for skilful editing of the manuscript.

REFERENCES

1. Y. Noma, P. Sideras, T. Naito, S. Bergstedt-Lindqvist, C. Azuma, E. Severinson, T. Tanabe, T. Kinashi, F. Matsuda, Y. Yaoita, and T. Honjo. Nature 319:640 (1986).
2. F. Lee, T. Yokota, T. Otsuka, P. Meyeson, D. Villaret, R. Coffman, T. Mosmann, D. Rennick, N. Roehm, C. Smith, A. Zlotnik, and K.-I. Arai. Proc. Natl. Acad. Sci. USA 83:2061 (1986).
3. T. Kinashi, N. Harada, E. Severinson, T. Tanabe, P. Sideras, M. Konishi, C. Azuma, A. Tominaga, S. Bergstedt-Lindqvist, M. Takahashi, F. Matsuda, Y. Yaoita, K. Takatsu, and T. Honjo. Nature 324:70 (1986).

4. T. Yokota, T. Otsuka, T. Mosmann, J. Banchereau, T. DeFrance, D. Blanchard, J.E. De Vries, F. Lee, and K.-I. Arai. Proc. Natl. Acad. Sci. USA 83:5894 (1986).
5. C. Azuma, T. Tanabe, M. Konishi, T. Kinashi, T. Noma, F. Matsuda, Y. Yaoita, K. Takatsu, L. Hammarström, C.I.E. Smith, E. Severinson, and T. Honjo. Nucl. Acids Res. 14:9149 (1986).
6. E. Severinson, P. Sideras, and S. Bergstedt-Lindqvist. Intern. Rev. Immunol. 2:143 (1987).
7. R. Fernandez-Boytran, P.H. Krammer, T. Diamantstein, J.W. Uhr, and E.S. Vitetta. J. Exp. Med. 164:580 (1986).
8. E. Severinson, T. Naito, H. Tokumoto, D. Fukushima, A. Hirano, K. Hama, and T. Honjo. Eur. J. Immunol. 17:67 (1987).
9. P. C. Isakson, E. Puré, E.S. Vitetta, and P.H. Krammer. J. Exp. Med. 155:734 (1982).
10. P. Sideras, S. Bergstedt-Lindqvist, H.R. MacDonald, and E. Severinson. Eur. J. Immunol. 15:586 (1985).
11. M. Howard, J. Farrar, M. Hilfiker, B. Johnson, K. Takatsu, T. Hamaoka, and W.E. Paul. J. Exp. Med. 155:914 (1982).
12. P. Sideras, K. Funa, I. Zalcberg-Quintana, K.G. Xanthopoulos, P. Kisielow, and R. Palacios. Proc. Natl. Acad. Sci. USA 85:218 (1988).
13. T. R. Mosmann, H. Cherwinski, M.W. Bond, M.A. Giedlin, and R.L. Coffman. J. Immunol. 136:2348 (1986).
14. S. N. Ho, R.T. Abraham, A. Nilson, B.S. Handwerger, and D.J. McKean. J. Immunol. 139:1532 (1987).
15. K. H. Grabstein, L.S. Park, P.J. Morrissey, H. Sassenfeld, V. Price, D.L. Urdal, and M.B. Widmer. J. Immunol. 139:1148 (1987).
16. N. Harada, M. Matsumoto, N. Koyama, A. Shimizu, T. Honjo, A. Tominaga, and K. Takatsu. Immunology Letters 17:1743 (1987).
17. E. Clutterbuck, J.G. Shields, J. Gordon, S.H. Smith, A. Boyd, R.E. Callard, H.D. Campbell, I.G. Young, and C.J. Sanderson. Eur. J. Immunol. 17:1743 (1987).
18. R. L. Coffman, J. Ohara, M.W. Bond, J. Carty, A. Zlotnik, and W.E. Paul. J. Immunol. 136:4538 (1986).
19. S. Bergstedt-Lindqvist, H.-B. Moon, U. Persson, G. Möller, C. Heusser, and E. Severinson. Eur. J. Immunol. 18:1073 (1988).
20. F. D. Finkelman, I.M. Katona, J.F. Urban, C.M. Snapper, J. Ohara, and W.E. Paul. Proc. Natl. Acad. Sci. USA 83:9675 (1986).
21. J. Stavnezer-Nordgren, and S. Sirlin. EMBO J. 5:95 (1986).
22. G. D. Yancopoulos, R.A. DePinho, K.A. Zimmerman, S.G. Lutzker, N. Rosenberg, and F.W. Alt. EMBO J. 5:3259 (1986).
23. M. R. Mowatt, and W.A. Dunnick. J. Immunol. 136:2674 (1986).
24. Y. Nishida, T. Kataoka, N. Ishida, S. Nakai, T. Kishimoto, I. Bottcher, and T. Honjo. Proc. Natl. Acad. Sci. USA 78:1581 (1981).

NORMAL AND ABNORMAL REGULATION OF HUMAN B CELL DIFFERENTIATION BY A NEW CYTOKINE, BSF2/IL-6

Tadamitsu Kishimoto, Tetsuya Taga, Katsuhiko Yamasaki, Tadashi Matsuda, Bo Tang, Atsushi Muraguchi, Yasuhiro Horii, Sachiko Suematsu, Yuichi Hirata, Hideo Yawata, Masatoshi Shimizu, Michiaki Kawano and Toshio Hirano

Institute for Molecular and Cellular Biology, Osaka University, 1-3 Yamadaoka, Suita, Osaka 565, Japan

Antibody molecules play an essential role not only in protection against viral or bacterial infections, but also in the induction of autoimmune diseases such as rheumatoid arthritis and systemic lupus erythematosus, and immediate-type hypersensitivity. Therefore, the study of the mechanism regulating the activation, proliferation and immunoglobulin secretion of B lymphocytes is essential for the normal and abnormal regulations in the antibody response.

It has been found that the differentiation of B cells into antibody producing cells is regulated by three distinct factors; i) BSF1/IL-4 for the activation of resting B cells, ii) BCGFII/IL-5 for the growth of activated B cells and iii) BSF2/IL-6 for the final maturation of B cells into antibody producing cells[1]. The cDNAs for these B cell factors (BSFs) have been cloned[2-5] and the presence and the involvement of BSFs in the process of B cell response have been confirmed. The studies with recombinant molecules, however, demonstrated that the functions of BSFs are not restricted to the B lineage cells but show a wide variety of biological functions[6]. One of the most typical examples is BSF2/IL-6; it shows growth and differentiation activities on a wide variety of tissues, such as on hepatocytes to induce acute phase proteins[7,8], on hematopoietic stem cells for their activation[9] and on T cells as a co-stimulatory factor for proliferation[10]. Therefore, BSF2/IL-6 may play a central role in host-defense mechanism(s).

HUMAN B CELL DIFFERENTIATION WITH BSF2/IL-6

B cell stimulatory factor 2 (BSF2) was originally identified as a factor which induces Ig-production in B lymphoblastoid cell lines or activated normal B cells[11,12]. The cDNA of IL-6 has been cloned and the nucleotide sequence and deduced amino acid sequence show that IL-6 consists of 212 amino acids including hydrophobic signal sequence with 28 amino acids (Fig. 1.A)[5]. Therefore, a secreted IL-6 consists of 184 amino acids with two possible N-glycosylation sites. A comparison of the amino acid sequence between human and murine IL-6 demonstrated that 10 amino acids between the residues 56 and 65 are identical and the positions of 4 cysteine residues are also conserved (Fig. 1.B). Thus, as shown in Fig. 1.B, this portion of IL-6 protein may have an essential role in the expression of IL-6 activity.

The cDNA of IL-6 was expressed in E. coli and recombinant IL-6 was purified as described[13]. The effect of rIL-6 on B cell response was studied. Human peripheral mononuclear cells (MNC) were cultured with varying concentrations of pokeweed mitogen (PWM) in the presence or absence of rIL-6. As shown in Fig. 2, the addition of rIL-6 markedly augmented the induction of IgM, IgG and IgA. However, rIL-6 did not show any effect on PWM-induced proliferation of peripheral MNC, indicating that IL-6 is a differentiation factor but not a growth factor for activated B cells[14].

In order to study whether IL-6 is essential for the Ig-induction in B cells, the effect of anti-IL-6 antibody was examined. Peripheral MNC were stimulated with PWM in the presence or absence of various concentrations of anti-IL-6. As shown in Fig. 3, 50 μg/ml anti-IL-6 antibody almost completely inhibited the PWM-induced Ig-production in B cells. $F(ab')_2$ fragments of anti-IL-6 antibody was also effective and the addition of rIL-6 could rescue the inhibitory effect of anti-IL-6, indicating that the neutralization of IL-6 with anti-IL-6 could inhibit Ig-induction in B cells. On the other hand, the same concentration of anti-IL-6 antibody did not show any inhibitory effect on PWM-induced proliferation of B cells, showing that IL-6 is essential for the Ig-induction but not required for the proliferation of B cells.

BSF2/IL-6 DOES NOT BELONG TO THE INTERFERON FAMILY

The cDNAs of interferon ß2 (IFNß2)[15] and 26 Kd protein[16] have been cloned and the results indicated that these molecules are identical with IL-6. IFNß2 was reported to have anti-viral activity and to be related to IFNß, based on the neutralization of its anti-viral activity by anti-IFNß[17]. It was, however, controversial whether IFNß2 is an IFN, since 26 Kd protein did not show any interferon

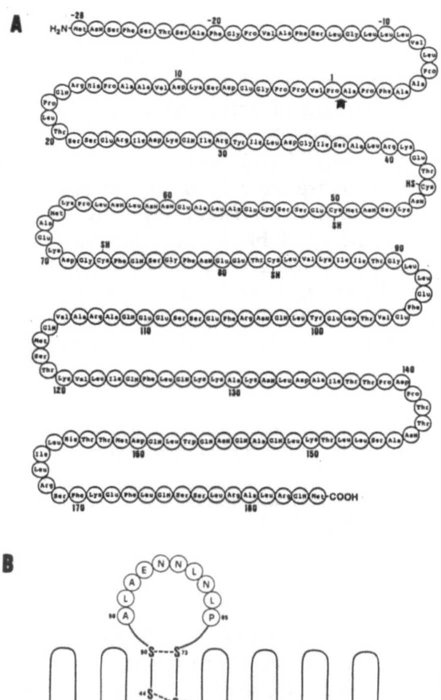

Fig. 1. A. Primary structure of human BSF2/IL-6
B. Amino acid residues between 56 and 65 are identical with murine BSF2/IL-6

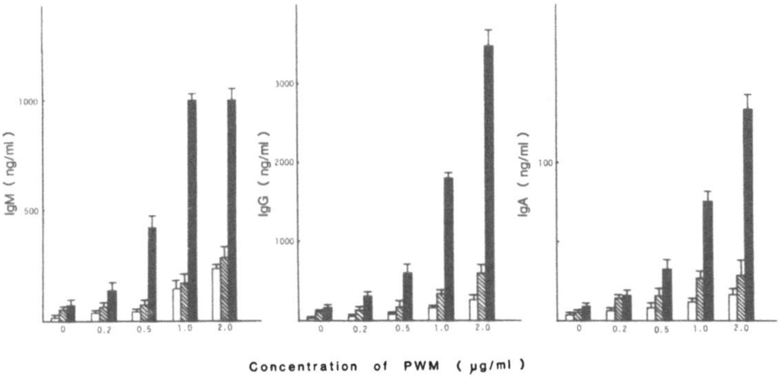

Fig. 2: Augmentation of Igs production in PWM-stimulated MNC.
: ☐ no BSF2/IL-6, ▧ : 1 ng/ml of BSF2/IL-6, ■ : 10 ng/ml of BSF2/IL-6

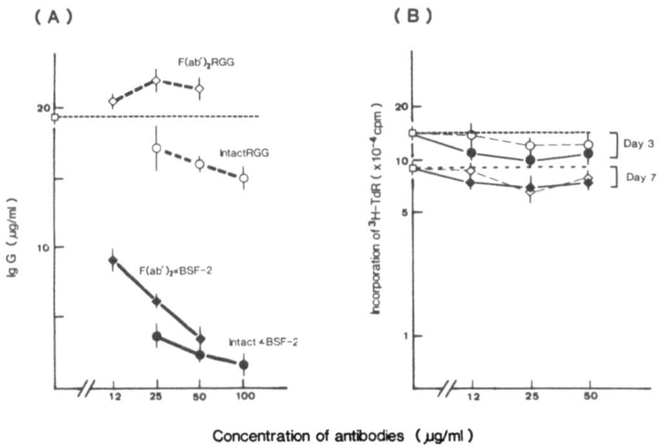

Fig. 3. Inhibition of PWM-induced Ig-production (A), but not proliferation (B), by anti-BSF2/IL-6 antibodies.

activity[18]. Thus, we tested anti-viral activity of rIL-6. The result clearly showed that rIL-6 did not have any anti-viral activity. Furthermore, anti-IFNß did not neutralize the activity of rIL-6 to induce Ig-production in B cells and anti-IL-6 did not neutralize the interferon activity of IFNß. These results indicate that IL-6 is functionally and immunologically not related to IFNs.

BSF2/IL-6 FUNCTIONS AS AN AUTOCRINE GROWTH FACTOR FOR MULTIPLE MYELOMA

The determination of N-terminal amino acid sequence of human myeloma growth factor indicated that IL-6 is identical with a myeloma growth factor[19]. The result suggests that abnormal expression of IL-6 may be related to the oncogenesis of human

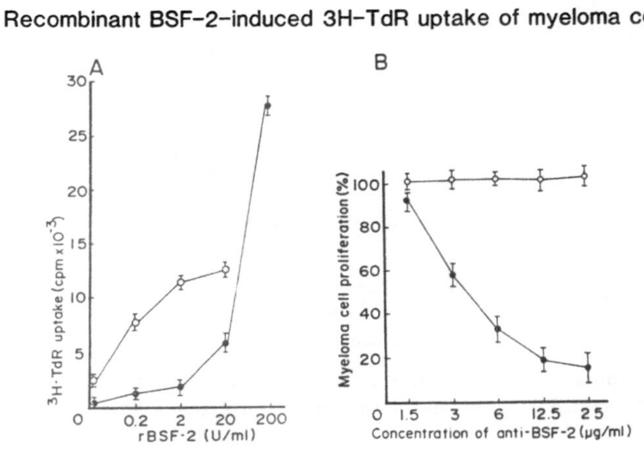

Fig. 4. (A) Augmentation of the proliferation of myeloma cells isolated from patients with multiple myeloma. Two representative cases are shown. (B) Neutralization of the activity of partially purified "myeloma growth factor" by anti-BSF2/IL-6 antibody.

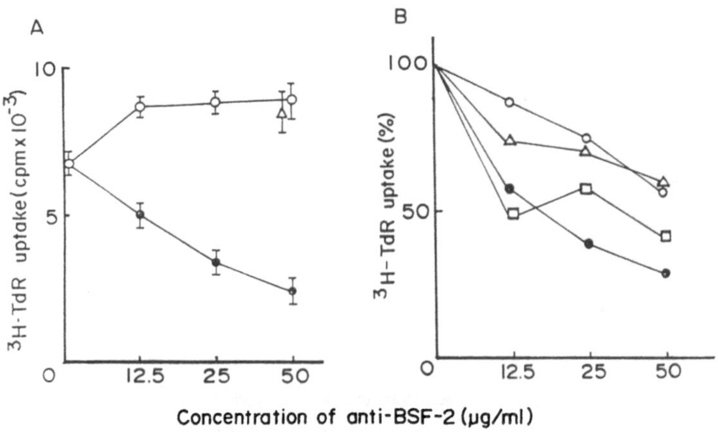

Fig. 5. (A) Inhibition of the in vitro growth of myeloma cells by anti-BSF2/IL-6 antibody (•—•) and the rescue of the inhibitory effect by the addition of rBSF2/IL-6 (o—o). (B) Inhibition of the growth in several different cases.

myelomas. Thus, we tested whether i) IL-6 can augment the proliferation of myeloma cells freshly isolated from patients, ii) myeloma cells produce IL-6 and iii) anti-IL-6 can inhibit the proliferation of myeloma cells. The results with myeloma cells isolated from 26 cases of myeloma patients indicated that IL-6 is indeed an autocrine growth factor for myeloma cells[20]. Thus, i) in 12 out of 26 cases, rIL-6 could augment the in vitro proliferation of myeloma cells (Fig. 4), ii) in all cases, myeloma cells constitutively expressed IL-6 mRNA, iii) the Scatchard plot analysis with ^{125}I-labelled IL-6 showed the expression of IL-6 receptor on all myeloma cells tested, and iv) most importantly, anti-IL-6 antibody could inhibit the in vitro proliferation of myeloma cells, as shown in Fig. 5. The result implicates that specific inhibitors of IL-6 or anti-IL-6 antibodies may be possible candidates for the specific therapy of multiple myelomas.

PLEIOTROPIC FUNCTIONS OF BSF2/IL-6

Infections, inflammations and tissue injuries induce disturbance of the physiological homeostasis and lead to a complex series of local and systemic reactions designated as acute phase response. The acute phase reaction is characterized by drastic changes in the levels of various plasma proteins, the so-called acute phase proteins, which are produced by the liver. The acute phase reaction is mediated by a factor tentatively called hepatocyte stimulating factor (HSF), which is mainly secreted from monocytes. IL-1 and TNF have been extensively studied as possible candidates inducing acute phase reactions. However, the studies with recombinant molecules have shown that those cytokines could induce only a limited acute phase reaction.

Recent studies with rIL-6 and anti-IL-6 antibodies[7, 8] clearly show that HSF is functionally and immunologically identical with IL-6. A rat hepatoma cell line (Foa-9) was incubated with various concentrations of rIL-6. rIL-6 induced a 5-fold increase in ß-fibrinogen mRNA level 12 hr after incubation. At the same time, albumin mRNA decreased 4 fold, indicating that rIL-6 induced acute phase reaction in the rat hepatoma cells. Furthermore, HSF activity present in conditioned medium from human monocytes was neutralized by anti-IL-6 antibodies. rIL-6 induced increases not only in ß-fibrinogen mRNA level but also in α_2-macroglobulin and cysteine proteinase inhibitor mRNA levels, but rIL-1 or TNF did not induce any increases in these acute phase proteins.

Thus, IL-6 is a cytokine which regulates the antibody response and acute phase reactions. IL-6 also acts on T cells, hematopoietic stem cells and nerve cells. It has been shown that IL-6 has a costimulatory activity for the proliferation of mitogen-stimulated T cells[10]. IL-6 is also responsible for the activation of hematopoietic stem cells to be responsive to IL-3[9].

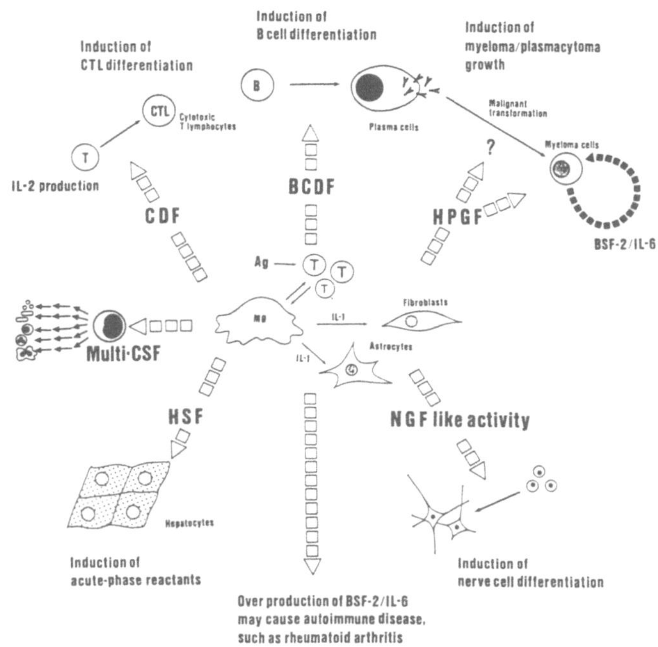

Fig. 6. Pleiotropic function of BSF2/IL-6

Stimulation of glioblastoma cells or astrocytoma cells with IL-1 induces IL-6 expression[21]. As IL-1 can be produced by glia cells, the result suggests that IL-6 may have a certain function in the brain. The study done by Satoh et al. (submitted) showed that IL-6 could induce the differentiation of a rat pheochromocytoma cell line into neuron cells, suggesting a certain activity of IL-6 on nerve cells. Thus, as summarized in Fig. 6, IL-6 shows a wide variety of biological functions on various tissues.

OVERPRODUCTION OF BSF2/IL-6 AND AUTOIMMUNE DISEASES

Systemic autoimmune diseases are characterized by hyperactivation of B cells and the production of various autoantibodies. Several studies in murine systems suggest that the dysregulation of lymphokine production or the production of abnormal lymphokines could be responsible for the hyperactivation of auto-antibody producing B cells. Since IL-6 is responsible for Ig-induction in B cells, IL-6 may be a principle lymphokine for generalized autoimmune diseases.

One of the typical examples is cardiac myxoma, which is a benign intraatrial heart tumor and one-third of the patients show autoimmune phenomenon with auto-antibody production. The culture supernatants of cardiac myxoma cells were found to display high IL-6 activity[22]. Northern blot analysis with the cDNA for IL-6 confirmed the elevated expression of mRNA in cardiac myxoma cells[5]. A similar situation was found in a patient with cervical cancer, who showed Sjögren-like syndrome and high titers of autoantibodies in the serum[22]. The tumor cells secreted large amounts of IL-6 and the patient's autoimmune symptoms disappeared 3 months after the surgical removal of the tumor. All these results strongly suggest that the overproduction of IL-6 may be responsible for autoantibody production and autoimmune phenomenon.

Then, the question to be asked is whether the overproduction of IL-6 is involved in the pathogenesis of generalized autoimmune diseases, such as rheumatoid arthritis (RA). The concentration of IL-6 in the synovial fluids from the affected joints of RA and OA (osteoarthritis) patients was measured by a RIA with anti-IL-6 antibodies. Both patients with affected joints contained excess synovial fluid. The result showed that 22 out of 25 specimens (92%) from RA patients showed detectable levels of IL-6. The mean value of IL-6 in these 22 samples was 15.6 ± 13 ng/ml (2.6 - 59 ng/ml). However, only 4 out of 17 specimens (24%) obtained from OA patients displayed detectable but low level of IL-6 (3.4 - 5.8 ng/ml). The synovial tissues (18 samples) biopsied from active RA patients, when incubated for 24 hr, produced large amounts of IL-6 (mean value was 212 ± 165 units/ml), and the activity was completely neutralized by anti-IL-6 antibodies. These results suggest that the unregulated productions of IL-6 may play an important role in the pathogenesis of RA and explain the infiltration of synovium by a large number of plasma cells and the production of various autoantibodies including rheumatoid factor. As it was described, IL-6 functions as hepatocyte stimulating factor to induce acute phase proteins and it also induces fever as an endogenous pyrogen[23]. Therefore, not only local but also several of the generalized symptoms in RA patients, such as hyper γ-globulinemia, an increase in acute phase proteins and fever, could be explained by the overproduction of IL-6.

HIGH AND LOW AFFINITY RECEPTORS FOR BSF2/IL-6

IL-6 receptor (IL-6-R) was studied using radioiodinated rIL-6 with a specific activity of 6×10^{13} cpm/g. Binding of ^{125}I-IL-6 to B lymphoblastoid cells, CESS, was competitively inhibited by unlabeled IL-6 but not by IL-1, IL-2, IFN-ß, IFN-γ and G-CSF, indicating the presence of receptors specific for IL-6[24].
EBV-transformed B lymphoblastoid cell lines expressed IL-6-R, but Burkitt's lines did not. The plasmacytoma cell lines and a hepatocyte cell line expressed IL-6-R, fitting the function of BSF2/IL-6 as a myeloma growth factor and a hepatocyte stimulating factor. The maximum number of IL-6-R was expressed on μ^+/δ^- activated B cells,

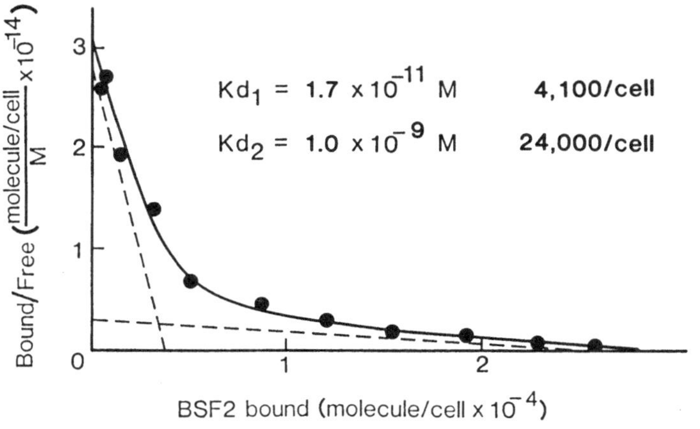

Fig. 7. Scatchard plot analysis of BSF2-R/IL-6 expressed on a myeloma cell line, U266

fitting the function of IL-6, which acts on B cells at the final maturation stage to induce immunoglobulin production.

Scatchard plot analysis of IL-6-R on a myeloma cell line, U266, demonstrated that both high and low affinity receptors with Kd value 1.7×10^{-11} and 1×10^{-9}M, respectively, were present on myeloma cells as shown in Fig. 7. The number of the receptors with higher affinity was about 10% of the total receptors.

MOLECULAR CLONING OF THE cDNA FOR THE BSF2/IL-6 RECEPTORS

In order to reveal the molecular structure of the IL-6-R and analyze the mechanism of signal transduction, attempts were made to clone the cDNA for the IL-6-R. The number of the IL-6-R expressed on the target cells was too small to prepare monoclonal antibodies against the receptor, usually in the order of 10^3/cell, and the situation is similar with other cytokine receptors. Therefore, fluorescein-conjugated IL-6 was employed as a probe for the detection of the IL-6-R. We also employed a high efficiency COS cell expression system with CDM8 vector, which was kindly provided by Dr. B. Seed (MGH).

A cDNA clone (pBSF2R.236) was isolated and the DNA was transfected into a murine fibroblast line, COP and transiently expressed. A portion of cells transfected with the DNA from a cDNA clone (pBSF2R.236) were positively stained with biotin-BSF2 and avidin-fluorescein, and the positive staining was inhibited by excess amount of non-labeled IL-6 but not by excess amount of IL-1 or IL-2, indicating that this cDNA clone (pBSF2R.236) includes the entire coding sequence of the IL-6-R. Scatchard plot analysis showed that COP cells transfected with the cDNA expressed a single homogenous receptor of lower affinity with the Kd value of 1×10^{-9}M. Northern blot analysis with the cDNA (pBSF2R.236) showed that mRNA of approximately 6 Kb was expressed in a myeloma cell line (U266), a B lymphoblastoid cell line (CESS) and a histiocytic cell line (U937) but not in a Burkitt's cell line (BL29) and a T cell line (Jurkat). The result coincided with the data obtained by the binding study.

As shown in Fig. 8, the nucleotide sequence and deduced amino acid sequence of the cDNA for IL-6-R demonstrates a typical membrane protein with signal peptide and transmembrane domain. The sequence does not show homology with any other protein and intracytoplasmic portion does not have tyrosine kinase domain.

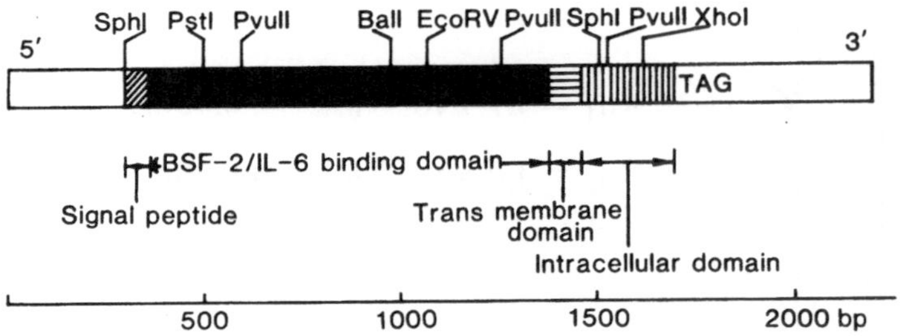

Fig. 8. Molecular structure of IL-6-R

CONCLUSION

The present studies demonstrate that BSF2/IL-6 has a wide variety of biological functions not only on activated B cells but also on T cells, hematopoietic stem cells, hepatocytes and nerve cells. Thus, BSF2/IL-6 may play a central regulatory role in host-defense mechanisms against infections, inflammations and tissue injuries. The studies also show that BSF2/IL-6 can be expressed in various tissues, such as T cells, monocytes, glial cells, fibroblasts, endothelial cells (Lotz et al., submitted), keratinocytes (unpublished) and various cancer cells, and it has been suggested that the abnormal expression of BSF2/IL-6 and the mechanism of signal transduction through the receptor molecules will provide critical information on the regulation of growth and differentiation of various cell types, and it will also shed light on the mechanism of pathogenesis of various diseases. Furthermore, it will provide new diagnostic means and treatment approaches to these diseases.

REFERENCES

1. T. Kishimoto, Factors affecting B-cell growth and differentiation, Ann. Rev. Immunol. 3:133 (1985).
2. Y. Noma, T. Sideras, T. NAito, A. Bergstedt-Lindqvist, C. Azuma, E. Severinson, T. Tanabe, T. Kinashi, F. Matsuda, Y. Yaoita, and T. Honjo, Cloning of cDNA encoding the murine IgG1 induction factor by a novel strategy using SP6 promoter. Nature 319:640 (1986).
3. F. Lee, T. Yokota, T. Otsuka, P. Meyerson, D. Villaret, N. Rocham, C. Smith, A. Zlotnick, and K. Arai, Isolation and characterization of a mouse interleukin cDNA clone that expresses B-cell stimulatory factor 1 activities and T-cell and mast cell-stimulating activities. Proc. Natl. Acad. Sci., USA 83:2061 (1986).
4. T. Kinashi, N. Harada, E. Severinson, R. Tanabe, P. Sideras, M. Konishi, C. Azuma, A. Tominaga, S. Bergstedt-Lindqvist, M. Takahashi, F. Matsuda, Y. Yaoita, K. Takatsu, and T. Honjo, Cloning of complementary DNA encoding T-cell replacing factor and identity with B-cell growth factor II. Nature 324:70 (1986).
5. T. Hirano, K. Yasukawa, H. Harada, T. Taga, Y. Watanabe, T. Matsuda, S. Kashiwamura, K. Nakajima, K. Koyama, A. Iwamatsu, S. Tsunasawa, F. Sakiyama, H. Matsui, Y. Takahara, T. Taniguchi, and T. Kishimoto, Complementary DNA for a novel human interleukin (BSF-2) that induces B lymphocytes to produce immunoglobulin. Nature 324:73 (1986).
6. T. Kishimoto and T. Hirano, Molecular regulation of B lymphocyte response. Ann. Rev. Immunol. 6:485 (1988).
7. J. Gauldie, C. Richards, D. Harnish, P. Lansdorp, and H. Baumann, Interferon ß2/BSF-2 shares identity with monocyte derived hepatocyte stimulating factor (HSF) and regulates the major acute phase protein response in liver cells. Proc. Natl. Acad. Sci., USA., in press (1987).

8. T. Andus, T. Geiger, T. Hirano, H. Northoff, U. Ganter, J. Bauer, T. Kishimoto, and P.C. Heinrich, Recombinant human B cell stimulatory factor 2 (BSF-2/INFß2) regulates ß-fibrinogen and albumin mRNA levels in Fa0-9 cells. FEBS Lett. 221:18 (1987)
9. K. Ikebuchi, G.G. Wong, S.C. Clark, J.N. Ihle, Y. Hirai, and M. Ogawa, Interleukin-6 enhancement of interleukin-3-dependent proliferation of multipotential hemopoietic progenitors. Proc. Natl. Acad. Sci., USA 84:9035 (1987).
10. M. Lotz, F. Jirik, R. Kabouridis, C. Tsoukas, T. Hirano, T. Kishimoto, and D.A. Carson. BSF-2/IL-6 is a costimulant for human thymocytes and T lymphocytes. J. Exp. Med, in press (1988).
11. A. Muraguchi, T. Kishimoto, Y. Miki, T. Kuritani, T. Kaieda, K. Yoshizaki, and Y. Yamamura, T cell-replacing factor (TRF)-induced IgG secretion in human B blastoid cell line and demonstration of acceptors for TRF. J. Immunol. 127:412 (1981).
12. T. Hirano, T. Taga, N. Nakano, K. Yasukawa, S. Kashiwamura, K. Shimuzu, K. Nakajima, K.H. Pyun, and T. Kishimoto, Purification to homogeneity and characterization of human B cell differentiation factor (BCDF or BSFp-2). Proc. Natl. Acad. Sci., USA. 82:5490 (1985).
13. T. Hirano, T. Matsuda, K. Hosoi, A. Okano, H. Matsui, and T. Kishimoto, Absence of antiviral activity in recombinant B cell stimulatory factor 2 (BSF-2). Immunol. Lett. 17:41 (1988).
14. A. Muraguchi, T. Hirano, B. Tang, T. Matsuda, Y. Horii, K. Nakajima, and T. Kishimoto, The essential role of B cell stimulatory factor 2 (BSF-2/IL-6) for the terminal differentiation of B cells. J. Exp. Med. 167:332 (1988).
15. A. Zilberstein, R. Ruggieri, J.H. Korn, and M. Revel, Structure and expression of cDNA and genes for human interferon-beta-2, a distinct species inducible by growth-stimulatory cytokines. EMBO Journal 5:2529 (1986).
16. G. Haegeman, J. Content, G. Volckaert, R. Derynck, J. Tavernieir, and W. Fiers, Structural analysis of the sequence encoding for an inducible 26-kDa protein in human fibroblasts. Eur. J. Biochem. 159: 625 (1986).
17. J. Weissenbach, Y. Chernajovsky, M. Zeevi, L. Shulman, H. Soreq, U. Nir, D. Wallach, M. Perricaudet, P. Tiollais, and M. Revel, Two interferon mRNA in human fibroblasts: In vitro translation and Escherichia coli cloning studies. Proc. Natl. Acad. Sci., USA. 77:7152 (1980).
18. P. Poupart, P. Vandenabeele, S. Cayphas, J.V. Snick, G. Haegeman, V. Kruys, W. Fiers, and J. Content, B cell growth modulating and differentiating activity of recombinant human 26-kd protein (BSF-2, HuIFN-ß2, HPGF). EMBO J. 6:1219 (1987).
19. J. Van Damme, G. Opdenakker, R.J. Simpson, M.R. Rubira, S. Cayphas, A. Vink, A. Billiau, and J. Van Snick, Identification of the human 26-kD protein, interferon ß2 (IFN-ß2), as a B cell hybridoma/plasmacytoma growth factor induced by interleukin 1 and tumor necrosis factor. J. Exp. Med. 165:914 (1987).
20. M. Kawano, T. Hirano, T. Matsuda, T. Taga, Y. Horii, K. Iwato, H. Asaoku, B. Tang, O. Tanabe, H. Tanaka, A. Kuramoto, and T. Kishimoto, Autocrine generation and essential requirement of BSF-2/IL-6 for human multiple myelomas. Nature, in press (1988).
21. K. Yasukawa, T. Hirano, Y. Watanabe, K. Muratani, T. Matsuda, S. Nakai, and T. Kishimoto, Structure and expression of human B cell stimulatory factor 2 (BSF-2) gene. EMBO J. 6:2939 (1987).
22. T. Hirano, T. Taga, K. Yasukawa, K. Nakajima, N. Nakano, F. Takatsuki, M. Shimuzu, A. Murashima, S. Tsunasawa, F. Sakiyama, and T. Kishimoto, Human B cell differentiation factor defined by an antipeptide antibody and its possible role in autoantibody production. Proc. Natl. Acad. Sci., USA. 84:228 (1987).
23. M.W. Nijsten, E.R. DeGroot, H.J. Duis, C.E. Hack, and L.A. Aarcen, Serum levels of interleukin 6 and acute phase response. Lancet ii: 921 (1987).
24. T. Taga, Y. Kawanishi, R.R. Hardy, T. Hirano, and T. Kishimoto, Receptors for B cell stimulatory factor 2 (BSF2): Quantitation, specificity, distribution and

ALTERNATIVE CYTOKINES IN THE IMMUNOREGULATION OF THE HUMAN B CELL CYCLE

John H. Kehrl and Anthony S. Fauci

Laboratory of Immunoregulation
National Institute of Allergy and Infectious Diseases
National Institutes of Health
Bethesda, MD 20892

INTRODUCTION

A variety of soluble factors have been described which regulate the growth and differentiation of human B lymphocytes in vitro. Several of these factors were orginally recognized by their activity in assays of B cell function, for example IL-4, BSF-2, and BCGF.[1-4] In contrast, we have been studying the effects on B cell function of three factors originally described to influence the function of cell types distinct from B cells. These three factors are Transforming Growth Factor-beta (TGF-ß), orginally described to induce certain adherent non-neoplastic cells to express a transformed phenotype and to undergo anchorage independent growth[5]; interleukin-2 (IL-2), first recognized to promote the growth of T lymphocytes[6]; and Tumor necrosis factors, first identified by their cytotoxic or cytostatic effects against certain tumor cell lines.[7] Each of these factors have been found to have significant regulatory effects on the growth and differentiation of human B cells in vitro.

TGF-ß

TGF-ß is a homodimeric protein first purified from human platelets, bovine kidney, and human placenta.[8-10] It has been partially sequenced and a cDNA has been cloned by recombinant DNA techniques.[11] TGF-ß exists in two molecular forms, TGF-ß1 and TGF-ß2, both homodimers of 112 amino acids per chain.[12,13] TGF-ß has been shown to act on a wide variety of cell types (reviewed M. B. Sporn et al.,[14]) and there is increasing evidence that TGF-ß may have an important role in the regulation of the immune system. TGF-ß1 has been shown to inhibit B and T cell proliferation[15,16]; inhibit natural killer cell activity[17]; inhibit the terminal differentiation of B cells to Ig secreting cells and the acquistion of kappa light chain by pre-B cells[15,18]; and to inhibit the generation of cytotoxic T cells.[19] Additionally, lymphoid cells have been shown to synthesize and secrete TGF-ß1.[15,16]

Besides TGF-ß1, TGF-ß2 also inhibits the proliferation of activated human B cells. The two molecular forms are equally potent in their inhibition of B cell DNA synthesis (Table 1). Besides their inhibition of growth factor dependent proliferation, TGF-ß1 and TGF-ß2 also inhibit the proliferation of resting B cells stimulated with a variety of activation signals; anti-mu plus BCGF, SAC, and phorbol myristate acetate plus ionomycin. PMA plus ionomycin is particularly sensitive to the inhibitory effects of TGF-ß. A series of studies have demonstrated that TGF-ß1 and TGF-ß2 inhibit B cell proliferation predominantly by inhibiting the G1 to S phase transition in the B cell cycle and not by

Table 1. TGF-ß1 and TGF-ß2 Inhibit the Proliferation of Activated B Cells in Response to IL-2 [1]

	DNA Synthesis (CPM)	
TGF-ß (ng/ml)	TGF-ß1	TGF-ß2
0	18,554	18,402
.015	16,430	18,662
.06	11,418	16,170
.025	7,613	8,512
1.0	4,546	4,939
4.0	1,767	2,728

[1]Two day activated B cells were cultured with 200 units per ml of recombinant IL-2 in the presence or absence of TGF-ß1 or TGF-ß2. ^{3}H-thymidine incorporation was measured during an 18 hr pulse 4 days later.

interfering with the early phases of B cell activation (J. H. Kehrl, manuscript in preparation).

In contrast, to its effect on normal B cell proliferation TGF-ß has been found to either have no effect or to enhance the proliferation of a variety of B cell lines. Blomhoff et al.[20] have presented evidence to suggest that infection with the Epstein-Barr Virus (EBV) may mediate a switch in responsiveness to TGF-ß. The growth of an EBV negative Burkitt's lymphoma cell line, normally unresponsive to TGF-ß, was stimulated by TGF-ß when the cell line was infected with the EBV virus. Similarly, we have found several EBV transformed B cell lines whose growth is stimulated by TGF-ß (unpublished observations). Additionally, a BCGF responsive B lymphoma cell line has been found which behaves like normal B cells in that it response to BCGF is inhibited by TGF-ß1 and TGF-ß2 (J. H. Kehrl et. al., manuscript in preparation). The cell line was found to express 5 fold more high affinity TGF-ß receptors than normal B cells plus a large number of low affinity receptors. Studies are in progress to further characterize the response of this cell line to TGF-ß and to examine the TGF-ß receptor on it in further detail.

Besides inhibiting B cell proliferation TGF-ß profoundly inhibits B cell Ig secretion. As with B cell proliferation both TGF-ß1 and TGF-ß2 are equally potent inhibitors of B cell differentiation (Table 2). TGF-ß inhibits not only the secretion of Ig but in addition the synthesis of Ig. ^{35}S labelling of B cells in the presence of TGF-ß and immunoprecipitation of the Ig revealed a marked reduction in both light chain and mu heavy chain synthesis (unpublished observation). Studies are in progress to confirm this observation at the mRNA level. Despite the inhibition of normal B cell differentiation TGF-ß has little or no effect on Ig production by EBV transformed B cell lines.[13] The reasons for this are unclear but may be related to the aberrant proliferative reponse these cell lines have to TGF-ß.

Although activated B and T cells would appear to synthesize TGF-ß in sufficient quantities to regulate their own proliferation and differentiation most cells including lymphocytes secrete predominantly an inert form of TGF-ß.[21,22] The biologically inert form of TGF-ß can be activated by exposure to acid (the purification of TGF-ß routinely involves an acidification step), by exposure to urea, by boiling for 3 minutes, or by exposure to certain proteases.[23] In order to address the question whether human B cells secrete sufficient active TGF-ß to regulate their own proliferation and differentiation, a series of experiments using an anti-sera which neutralizes the active but not the inert form of TGF-ß1 were performed. The addition of the anti-sera to B cell cultures had little effect on levels of B cell DNA synthesis although in an occasional

Table 2. Inhibits the Differentiation of Human B Lymphocytes to Ig Secretion [1]

TGF-ß2 (ng/ml)	IgG (ng/ml)	IgM (ng/ml)
0	1,880	4,480
.015	1,210	2,330
.0625	946	1,860
.025	355	860
1.0	192	230
4.0	170	540

[1]Two day activated B cells were cultured with 200 units per ml of recombinant IL-2 in the presence or absence of TGF-ß2. Supernatant IgG and IgM were measured 7 days later.

experiment there was a small enhancement. In contrast, in 9 of 10 experiments the antibody enhanced B cell Ig secretion when compared to the pre-immune antisera (J. H. Kehrl, manuscript in preparation). These findings suggest that sufficient active TGF-ß is endogenously produced to regulate B cell differentiation.

Finally, the observation that TNF-α could partially reverse the inhibitory effects of TGF-ß on the generation of cytotoxic T cells[19] prompted us to determine whether TNF-α might have a similar effect on TGF-ß's inhibition of B cell Ig production. Since we had previously observed that TNF-α enhanced B cell differentiation this was an attractive hypothesis; however, TNF-α was unable to reverse the inhibitory effects of TGF-ß (Table 3). The mechanisms by which TGF-ß inhibits B cell differentiation and whether this inhibition in reversible remains to be established.

Table 3. TNF-α Does not Reverse the Inhibitory Effects of TGF-ß on B Cell Ig Secretion[1]

Factors[2]	Experiment 1 IgM (ng/ml)	Experiment 2 IgM (ng/ml)
-	40	260
IL-2	960	1,460
IL-2 + TNF-α	1,200	3,220
IL-2 + TGF-ß	10	260
IL-2 + TNF-α + TGF-ß	10	400

[1]Activated B cells were cultured with the above factors for 7 days and supernatant IgG and IgM were obtained measured by an isotype specific ELISA.

[2]Factor concentrations were the following: IL-2 at 200 ng/ml, TNF-α at 50 units/ml, and TGF-ß at 2 ng/ml.

TUMOR NECROSIS FACTOR-ALPHA AND LYMPHOTOXIN

TNF-α and lymphotoxin are 17 and 21 kilodalton proteins, respectively, each originally described on the basis of their cytotoxic or cytostatic effects on certain tissue culture cell lines and on the growth of certain tumors in vivo.[6,24,25] Subsequently, each factor has been found to have a broad spectrum of biological activities affecting a variety of cell types (reviewed by Beutler and Cerami,[26]). The previous observations that certain monocyte/macrophage products influenced B cell function[27,28] and that a factor which triggered the selective diffentiation of murine B cells was present in the serum of LPS-treated Bacillus Calmette-Guerin (BCG)-infected mice[29] prompted us to examine the potential role of TNF-α in human B cell function. Of note, the serum of such treated mice causes hemmorrhagic necrosis of certain tumors in mice and that activity was the first description of TNF-α.[6]

Stimulation of human B cells with the polyclonal B cell activator, Staphylococcus aureus Cowan strain I (SAC), is only sufficient to trigger an initial round of B cell proliferation. However, the addition of an appropriate growth factor will prolong the proliferative response. This observation was the basis of the first assay for human BCGF.[30] The addition of TNF-α to SAC-activated B cells results in a prolongation of B cell DNA synthesis similar to BCGF.[31] The magnitiude of the response can be augmented by the addition of other factors such as IL-1 and interferon-gamma (figure 1). Additionally, TNF-α will augment the proliferative response triggered by IL-2. While TNF-α even in the presence of IL-1 or interferon-gamma will not induce significant Ig secretion by SAC-activated B cells, it will enhance the induction of Ig secretion by IL-2.[29]

After observing that TNF-α had significant effects upon B cell function we examined the effects of the structurally and functionally related protein, lymphotoxin.[32] The cloning of the cDNAs for TNF-α and lymphotoxin had previously revealed a 30% identity between the amino acid sequences, and competitive binding experiment with radiolabeled recombinant material had demonstrated that both proteins interact with the same receptor.[32,33] We found that similar to TNF-α, lymphotoxin also enhances human B cell proliferation and differentiation.[32] Since lymphotoxin is

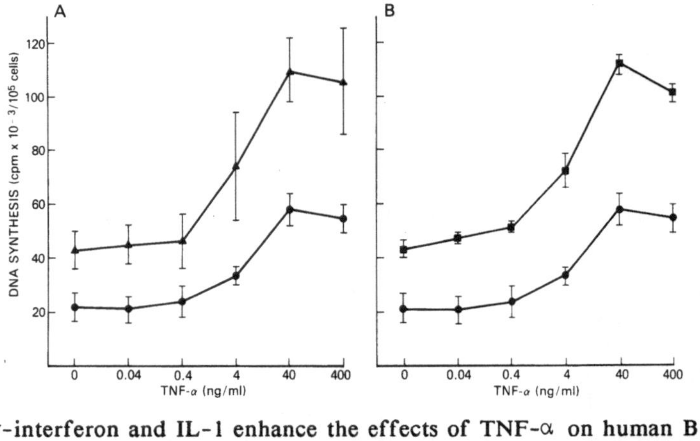

Fig. 1. γ-interferon and IL-1 enhance the effects of TNF-α on human B cell proliferation. 2 day activated B cells were cultured in the presence of increasing concentrations of TNF-α in the presence (▲---▲) or absence (•---•) of γ-interferon (100 u/ml) in part A and in the presence (■---■) or absence of (•---•) of IL-1 (10 u/ml) in part B. ^{3}[H]-thymidine incorporation was measured during the last 18 h of a 4 day culture.

predominantly a lymphocyte derived product we also asked the question whether lymphotoxin could account for part of the growth promoting activity found in crude supernatants derived from activated normal T cells.[32] Using a neutralizing antibody to lymphotoxin we were able to neutralize 70% of the growth promoting activity of a supernatant conditioned by PHA-activated T cells in the SAC assay for BCGF. The antibody had no inhibitory effect on IL-2 triggered proliferation and the inhibitory effects of the antibody could be reversed by an excess of recombinant lymphotoxin. Similarily we showed that much of the BCGF activity present in a commercially available preparation of BCGF could be accounted for by the presence of lymphotoxin.[32] These data implicated both TNF-α and lymphotoxin as important factors in the regulation of the humoral immune response in vivo.

Also, we have radiolabelled TNF-α and performed binding and chemical crosslinking studies with resting and activated B cells. TNF-α was radiolabelled with ^{125}I using a chloramine T method. The iodinated material runs as a single band on SDS-PAGE at

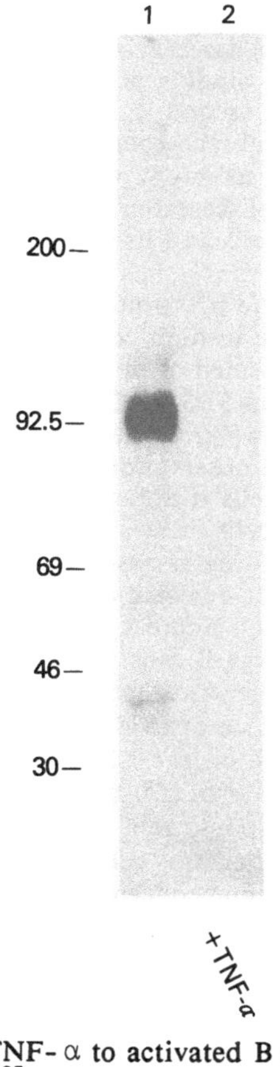

Fig. 2. Crosslinking of ^{125}I-TNF-α to activated B cells. 2 day activated B cells were incubated with ^{125}I-TNF-α (1nM) in the presence (lane 2) or absence (lane 1) of a 100 fold molar excess of unlabelled TNF-α. Following covalent linkage of ^{125}I-TNF-α to its plasma membrane receptor with disuccinimidyl suberate (DSS), the complex was immunoprecipitated with an anti-TNF-α antibody and analyzed by SDS-PAGE.

17kd. When the ^{125}I-TNF was used in radioreceptor binding assays, unactivated B cells were found to have undectable numbers of receptor. However, 2 day SAC activated B cells were found to have approximately 6000 receptors per cell with an estimated Kd of 200pM.[31] Lymphotoxin but not IL-1, IL-2, or interferon-gamma competitively inhibited the binding. These results with the activated B cells are consistent with results from binding assays performed with cell lines sensitive to the cytotoxic effects of TNF-α. When the ^{125}I-TNF is chemically crosslinked to the surface of SAC activated B cells and the crosslinked species examined by SDS-PAGE, a prominent band at 91 kD and 2 less prominent bands at 74 and 55 kD are visualized (figure 2). The addition of a 100 fold excess of unlabelled TNF-α blocked the detection of the complexes. These crosslinked species would correspond to 3 proteins of 74, 57, and 38 kD suggesting a multi-chain TNF-α/lymphotoxin receptor on human B cells. These results are consistent with results from other laboratories examining TNF-α receptors on other cell types.[34,35]

INTERLEUKIN-2

Since the first description of a T Cell Growth Factor, IL-2, there has been a controversy on whether IL-2 also influences either B cell growth or differentiation. Although there remain a few skeptics there is a general consensus that IL-2 has an important role in both B cell proliferation and B cell differentiation.[36,37] It will co-stimulate with anti-mu in the induction of B cell DNA synthesis, maintain the proliferation of SAC-activated B cells, and induce the differentiation of SAC-activated B cells to Ig secretion. More recently there has been data published suggesting that IL-2 may directly activate B cells via an IL-2 binding protein distinct from the Tac protein.[38] The recent identification of a second IL-2 binding protein distinct from the Tac protein which forms a membrane complex with the Tac protein to form a high affinity IL-2 receptor[39-43] has prompted us in conjunction with Warner Greene and Mitchell Dukovich at the Hughes Medical Research Institute, Duke University, to examine the expression of the p70 protein on B cells and its role in B cell function.

A recent study had suggested that the p70 protein was present on resting T cells and accounted for their proliferative response to high concentrations of IL-2.[44] Using highly purified tonsillar B cells we performed chemical crosslinking with ^{125}I-IL-2 and examined the crosslinked species with SDS-PAGE. We were unable to demonstrate the presence of the p70-IL-2 complex even when we attempted to immunoprecipitate the complex with an anti-IL-2 antibody (unpublished observation). Although this did not establish that p70 was not present on tonsillar B cells it did suggest that if it were present it was either on a small population of the cells or at a very low density. To address this question we performed radioreceptor binding assays with ^{125}I-IL-2 using size fractionated B cells. IL-2 binding was not detected on the small, presumably resting and non-cycling B cells. However, both a small number of high affinity and intermediate affinity receptors were present on the large B cells. The finding of intermediate affinity receptors on the large B cells suggested that they may express small amounts of p70 in the absence of Tac. One other piece of evidence which suggests that a population of B cells may express p70 in the absence of Tac is the observation that the lymphoblastoid B cell line, SKW.6B, expresses p70 but not Tac. This cell line was originally described to secrete IgM in response to a B cell differentiation factor.[45] Subsequently, it was observed that this cell line would secrete IgM when cultured in the presence of high but not low concentrations of IL-2.[46] Chemical crosslinking of ^{125}I-IL-2 to SKW6.B cells and analysis by SDS-PAGE revealed an 88 kD band consistent with p70 crosslinked to IL-2. Binding assays revealed approximately 900 receptors with an estimated Kd of 850 pm consistent with results obtained with other cell lines which expressed p70 in the absence of Tac.[43] These findings suggest that only the large tonsillar B cells are stimulated via high concentrations of IL-2 and that this stimulation likely occurs via the p70 molecule.

Similar to activated T cells activated B cells readily express the p70 protein in conjuction with the Tac protein. Two day SAC-activated B cells when chemically crosslinked to ^{125}I-IL-2 and analyzed by SDS-PAGE revealed a 70 kD band consistent

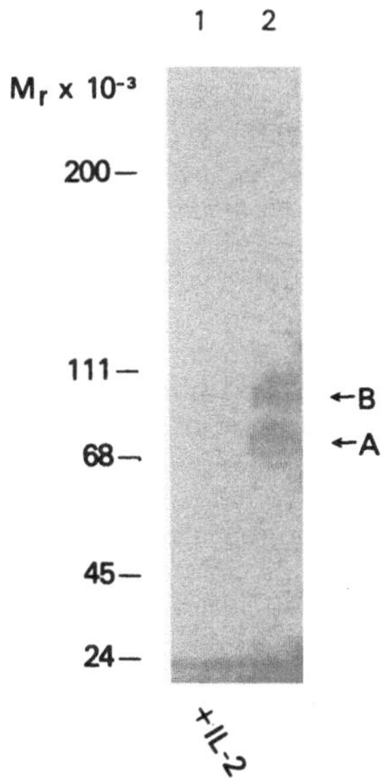

Fig. 3. Crosslinking of ^{125}I-IL-2 to activated B cells. 2 day SAC activated B cells were incubated with ^{125}I-IL-2 (200pM) in the presence (lane 1) or absence (lane 2) of a 100 fold excess of unlabelled IL-2. Following crosslinking with DSS a crude membrane preparation was made and analyzed by SDS-PAGE.

with the Tac protein crosslinked to IL-2 and a 88 kD band consistent with the P70 protein crosslinked to IL-2 (figure 3). The presence of non-radiolabelled IL-2 blocks detection of both bands. Thus, these data demonstrate that normal activated B cells are able to express both proteins known to be associated with high and low affinity IL-2 receptors and give further credence to the importance of IL-2 in the regulation of human B cell function.

CONCLUSIONS

Understanding the role of various soluble factors in human B cell activation, proliferation, and differentiation has become a progressively more complex issue. It is clear that there are a variety of soluble factors which enhance the growth and differentiation of B cells in vitro. The large number of factors which have been identifed to promote B cell proliferation and differentiation suggest considerable redundancy in the regulatory processes or it is possible that our crude assays of cellular function do not adequately assess the subtle differences between the various factors. In addition to their obvious effects on B cell growth and Ig production these factors may have other important effects on B cell function. Also, of note is the apparent lack of lineage specificity of many of the factors which were either originally identified as B cell specific factors, i.e IL-4 and BSF-2, and have been subsequently shown to effect other cell types or, conversely, factors such as TNF-α which were orginally identified by their effects on other cell types and have been subsequently shown to influence B cell function.

In contrast to the large number factors which have been shown to enhance B cell function there are relatively few well described negative regulatory factors. TGF-ß is perhaps the best characterized of these factors. Furthermore, TGF-ß is the only such factor to be shown to be secreted by B cells themselves implicating TGF-ß as a potential autoregulator of B cell function. Crucial to determining the role of TGF-ß as an autocrine regulator of B cell function will be an understanding of the mechanisms by which it is activated in vivo and the regulatory processes controlling its activation.

REFERENCES

1. W.E. Paul, and J. Ohara, B-cell stimulatory factor-1/interleukin 4. Annu. Rev. Immunol. 4:429 (1987).
2. T. Kishimoto, T. Hirano, H. Kikutani, and A. Muraguchi, Delineation of human B cell differentiation: immunological and molecular characterization of human B cell differentiation factor (BSF-2). Adv. Exp. Med. Biol. 213:177 (1987).
3. J.L. Butler, A. Muraguchi, H.C. Lane, and A.S. Fauci, Development of a human T-T cell hybridoma secreting B cell growth factor. J. Exp. Med. 157:60 (1983).
4. J.L. Ambrus, Jr., C.H. Jurgensen, E.J. Brown, and A.S. Fauci, Purification to homogeneity of a high molecular weight human B cell growth factor, demonstration of specific binding to activated B cells, and development of a monoclonal antibody to the factor. J. Exp. Med. 162:1319 (1985).
5. D.A. Morgan, F.W. Ruscetti, and R.C. Gallo, Selective in vitro growth of T lymphocytes from normal human bone marrows. Science. 193:1007 (1976).
6. E.A. Carswell, L.J. Old, R.L. Kassel, S. Green, N. Fiore, and B. Williamson, an endotoxin-induced serum factor that causes necrosis of tumors. Proc. Natl. Acad. Sci. USA. 72:3666 (1975).
7. A.B. Roberts, C.A. Frolik, M.A. Anzano, and M.B. Sporn, Transforming growth factors from neoplastic and nonneoplastic tissues. Fed. Proc. 42:2621 (1983).
8. R.K. Assoian, A. Komoriya, C.A. Meyers, and M.B. Sporn, Transforming growth factor-ß in human platelets: identification of a major storage site, purification, and characterization. J. Biol. Chem. 258:7155 (1983).
9. C.A. Frolik, L.L. Dart, C.A. Meyers, D.M. Smith, and M.B. Sporn, Purification and initial characterization of a type ß transforming growth factor from human placenta. Proc. Natl. Acad. Sci. USA. 80:3676 (1983).
10. A. Roberts, M. Anzano, C. Meyers, J. Wideman, R. Blacher, Y.E. Pan, S. Stein, S.R. Lehrman, J.M. Smith, L.C. Lamb, and M.B. Sporn, Purification and properties of a type ß transforming growth factor from bovine kidney. Biochemistry. 22:5692 (1983).
11. R. Derynck, J.A. Jarrett, E.Y. Chen, D.H. Eaton, J.R. Bell, R.K. Assoian, A.B. Roberts, M.B. Sporn, and D.V. Geoddel, Human transforming growth factor-ß complementary DNA sequence and expression in normal and transformed cells. Nature 316:701 (1985).
12. S. Cheifetz, J.A. Weatherbee, M.L.-S. Tsang, J.K. Anderson, J.E. Mole, R. Lucas, and J. Massagué, The transforming growth factor-ß system, a complex pattern of cross-reactive ligands and receptors. Cell. 48:409 (1987).
13. P.R. Seyedin, P.R. Segarini, D.M. Rosen, A.Y. Thompson, H. Bentz, and J. Graycor, Cartilage inducing factor-ß is a unique protein structurally and functionally related to transforming growth factor-ß. J. Biol. Chem. 262:1946 (1987).
14. A.B. Roberts, and M.B. Sporn, Transforming growth factor-ß. Adv. Cancer Res. 1988 in press.
15. J.H. Kehrl, L.M. Wakefield, A.B. Roberts, S. Jakowlew, M. Alvarez-Mon, R. Derynck, M.B. Sporn, and A.S. Fauci, Production of transforming growth factor-ß by human T lymphocytes and its potential role in the regulation of T cell growth. J. Exp. Med. 163:1037 (1986).
16. J.H. Kehrl, A.B. Roberts, L.M. Wakefield, S. Jakowlew, M.B. Sporn, and A.S.Fauci, Transforming growth factor-ß is an important immunomodulatory protein for human B lymphocytes. J. Immunol. 137:3855 (1987).
17. A.H. Rook, J.H. Kehrl, L.M. Wakefield, A.B. Roberts, M.B. Sporn, D.B. Burlington, H.C. Lane, and A.S. Fauci, Effects of transforming growth factor-ß on the functions of natural killer cells: depressed cytolytic activity and blunting of interferon responsiveness. J. Immunol. 136:3916 (1986).
18. G. Lee, L.R. Elingsworth, S. Gillis, R. Wall, and P.W. Kincade, ß-transforming growth factors are potential regulators of B lymphopoiesis. J. Exp. Med. 166:1290 (1987).
19. G.E. Ranges, I.S. Figari, T. Espevik, and M.A. Palladino, Jr., Inhibition of cytotoxic T cell development by transforming growth factor ß and reversal by recombinant tumor necrosis factor α. J. Exp. Med. 166:991 (1987).
20. H.K. Blomhoff, E. Smeland, A.S. Mustafa, T. Godal, and R. Ohlsson, Epstein-Barr virus mediates a switch in responsiveness to transforming growth factor, type ß, in cells of the B cell lineage, Eur. J. Immunol. 17:299 (1987).

21. D.A. Lawrence, R. Pircher, C. Kryceve-Martinerie, and P. Jullien, Normal embryo fibroblasts release transforming growth factors in a latent form. J. Cell. Physiol. 121:184 (1984).
22. R. Pircher, D.A. Lawrence, and P. Jullien, Latent ß-transforming growth factor in non-transformed and Kirsten sarcoma virus-transformed normal rat kidney cells. Cancer Res. 44:5538 (1984).
23. D.A. Lawrence, R. Pircher, and P. Jullien, Conversion of a high molecular weight latent ß-TGF from chicken embryo fibroblasts into a low molecular weight active ß-TGF under acidic conditions. Biochem. Biophys. Res. Comm. 133:1026 (1985).
24. D. Pennica, G.E. Nedwin, J.S. Hayflick, P.H. Seeburg, R. Derynck, M.A. Palladino, W.J. Kohr, B.B. aggarwal, and D.V. Goeddel, Human tumour necrosis factor: precursor structure, expression and homology to lymphotoxin. Nature. 312:724 (1984).
25. P.W. Gray, B.B. Aggarwal, C.V. Benton, T.S. Bringman, W.J. Henzel, J.A. Jarrett, D.W. Leung, B. Moffat, P. Ng, L.P. Svedersky, M.A. Palladino, and G.E. Nedwin, Cloning and expression of cDNa for human lymphotoxin, a lymphokine with tumor necrosis activity. Nature 312:721 (1984).
26. B. Beutler, A. Cerami, Cachectin and tumour necrosis factor as two sides of the same biological coin. Nature. 320:584 (1986).
27. R.J.M. Falkoff, J.L. Bulter, C.A. Dinarello, and A.S. Fauci, Direct effects of a monoclonal B cell differentiation factor and of purified interleukinn 1 on B cell differentiation. J. Immunol. 133:692 (1986).
28. M.K. Hoffmann, S. Koenig, R.S. Mittler, H.F. Oettgen, P. Ralph, C. Galanos, and U. Hammerling, Macrophge factor controlling differentiation of B cells. J. Immunol. 122:497 (1979).
29. M.K. Hoffmann, S. Green, L.J. Old, and H.F. Oettgen, Serum containing endotoxin-induced tumor necrosis factor substitutes for helper T cells. Nature. 263:416 (1976).
30. A. Muraguchi, and A.S. Fauci, Proliferative responses of normal human B lymphocytes. Development of an assay system for human B cell growth factor (BCGF). J. Immunol. 129:1104 (1982).
31. J.H. Kehrl, A. Miller, and A.S. Fauci, Effect of tumor necrosis factor α on mitogen-activated human B cells. J. Exp. Med. 166:786 (1987).
32. J.H. Kehrl, M. Alvarez-Mon, G.A. Delsing, and A.S. Fauci, Lymphotoxin is an important T cell-derived growth factor for human B cells. Science. 238:1144 (1987).
33. B.B. Aggarwal, T.E. Eessalu, P.E. Hass, Characterization of receptors for human tumour necrosis factor and their regulation by γ-IFN. Nature. 318:665 (1985).
34. P. Scheurich, U. Ucer, M. Kronke, and K. Pfizenmaier, Quantification and characterization of high affinity membrane receptors for tumor necrosis factor on human leukemic cell lines. Int. J. Cancer. 38:127 (1986).
35. A.A. Creasey, R. Yamamoto, and C.R. Vih, A high molecular weight component of the human tumor necrosis factor receptor is associated with cytotoxicity. Proc. Natl. Acad. Sci. USA. 84:3293 (1987).
36. A. Muraguchi, J.H. Kehrl, D.L. Longo, D.J. Volkman, and A.S. Fauci, Tac expression on activated B cells and on a human T-cell leukemia-infected B-cell line. J. Exp. Med. 161:181 (1985).
37. M. Tsudo, T. Uchiyama, and H. Uchino, Expression of Tac antigen on activated normal human B cells. J. Exp. Med. 160:602 (1984).
38. Le thi Bich-thuy and A.S. Fauci, Direct effect of interluekin 2 on the differentiation of human B cells which have not been preactivated in vitro. Eur. J. Immunol. 15:1075 (1985).
39. M. Sharon, R.D. Klausner, B.R. Cullen, R. Chizzonite, and W.J. Leonard, Novel IL-2 receptor subunit detected by cross-linking under high affiity conditions. Science. 234:859 (1986).
40. M. Tsudo, R.W. Kozak, C.K. Goldman, and T.A. Waldmann, Demonstration of a non-Tac peptide that binds interleukin 2: a potential participant in a multichain interleukin 2 receptor complex. Proc. Natl. Acad. Sci. USA. 83:9694 (1986).
41. K. Teshigawara, H. Wang, K. Kato, and K.A. Smith, Interleukin 2 high-affinity receptor expression requires two distinct binding protiens. J. Exp. Med. 165:223 (1987).
42. R.J. Robb, C.M. Rusk, J. Yodoi, W.C. Greene, An interleukin 2 binding molecule distinct from the Tac protein: analysis of its role in formation of high affinity receptors. Proc. Natl. Acad. Sci. USA. 84:2002 (1987).

43. M. Dukovich, Y. Wano, Le thi Bich-Thuy, P. Katz, B.R. Cullen, J.H. Kehrl, and W.C. Greene, Identification of a second human interluekin-2 binding protein and its role in the assembly of the high affinity IL-2 receptor. Nature. 327:518 (1987).
44. Le thi Bich-Thuy, M. Dukovich, N.J. Peffer, A.S. Fauci, J.H. Kehrl, and W.C. Greene, Direct activation of human T cells by IL-2: the role of an IL-2 receptor distinct from the Tac protein. J. Immunol. 239:1550 (1987).
45. P. Ralph, O. Saiki, D.H. Maurer, and K. Welte, IgM and IgG secretion in human B cell liens regulted by B cell-inducing factors (BIF) and phorbol ester. Immunol. Letter 7:17 (1983).
46. P. Ralph, G. Jeong, K. Welte, R. Mertelsmann, H. Rabin, L.E. Henderson, L.M. Souza, T.C. Boone, and R.J. Robb, Stimulation of immunoglobulin secretion in human B lymphocytes as a direct effect of high concentrations of IL-2. J. Immunol. 133:2442 (1984).

INDEX